RBTIOM Concepts and Principles

An **Original Medicine** Perspective on **RBTI**
(*Reams Biological Theory of Ionization*)

$$Ph = CS + 1.5 \; \frac{6.4}{6.4} \; 6.5C \; .04M \; \frac{3}{3}$$

World rights reserved. This book or any portion thereof may not be copied or reproduced in any form or manner whatever, except as provided by law, without the written permission of the authors, except by a reviewer who may quote brief passages in a review.

The author assumes full responsibility for the editing of and accuracy of all facts and quotations as cited in this book. The opinions expressed in this book are the author's personal views and interpretations, and do not necessarily reflect those of the publisher.

This book is provided with the understanding that the publisher is not engaged in giving spiritual, legal, medical, or other professional advice. If authoritative advice is needed, the reader should seek the counsel of a competent professional.

Copyright © 2024 Jim Sharps, N.D., H.D., Dr. NSc
Copyright © 2024 TEACH Services, Inc.
ISBN-13: 978-1-4796-1760-9 (Paperback)
ISBN-13: 978-1-4796-1786-9 (Spiral)
ISBN-13: 978-1-4796-1761-6 (ePub)
Library of Congress Control Number: 2024908292

For further information, contact:
International Institute of Original Medicine, P. O. Box 311, Smithfield, VA 23431
Or visit https://iiomonline.org/

Cover and Text Design: Elisa Ramirez-Sharps and Timothy J. Sharps

Edited by Betty Reams Hernandez

Printed by

www.TEACHServices.com • (800) 367-1844

Foreword

Original Medicine was developed by God and is written throughout the Holy Bible. It cannot be improved upon and is honored and taught by Seventh Day Adventist Medical Missionaries, as well as others who follow the tenets of Original Medicine in the Bible.

RBTI was developed by Carey A. Reams in 1931, while fasting and praying, in an effort to find a way to help a small child who was dying. Thus began 50 years of research and results that enabled Reams to design nutritional programs for plants, animals, and people.

In his later years, Dr. Reams taught others how to continue what he had started and traveled the US teaching RBTI classes in agriculture, animal husbandry, and human health. He worked up until the day that he died in 1985, carefully passing on his teachings to select students who had excelled.

Any good educator knows that a student receives teaching through his or her own perception, and as time went by, disagreements arose about who was right and who was wrong. And this was the state of affairs that I found in 2016 when RBTI appeared in social media. Many who were teaching were getting good results, but few were agreeing one with another.

The term, "Original Medicine," was not known to Carey Reams; however, he was a Seventh Day Adventist and a man whose love of God and life spoke for itself. If he were alive today, he would applaud the combination of RBTI and Original Medicine.

Original Medicine is God's law for human health. RBTI was given by God to Carey Reams, for the scientific, mathematical proof of HIS laws. Dr. Reams didn't use the words "Original Medicine," but he quoted the tenets right from the Bible, and he lived it in word and deed. I am certain we have his approval to call what we do RBTIOM!

Betty Reams Hernandez
RBTI Living, President and CEO

TABLE OF CONTENTS

Foreword iii
RBTIOM Preface 5
What is Original Medicine? 6
What is RBTI? 7
What is RBTIOM? 10
The Eight Laws of Health 12
    PURE AIR IS ESSENTIAL FOR RADIANT HEALTH 13
    PURE WATER IS ESSENTIAL FOR RADIANT HEALTH......................... 16
    SUNLIGHT IS ESSENTIAL FOR RADIANT HEALTH 19
    NUTRITION IS ESSENTIAL FOR RADIANT HEALTH............................. 21
    EXERCISE IS ESSENTIAL FOR RADIANT HEALTH 24
    Adequate Rest is Essential for Radiant Health....................................... 27
    Temperance is Essential for Radiant Health.. 31
    TRUST IN DIVINE POWER IS ESSENTIAL FOR RADIANT HEALTH 33
    Eight Laws of Health: SUMMARY AND CONCLUSIONS 37
    Final Thoughts on Original Medicine 38
    Summary and Conclusions 38
Basic Concepts and Explanation of RBTI 40
    Origin and Basics of RBTI 40
    The Mathematical Formula for Perfect Health... 42
    Summary of RBTI Analysis: 44
    Ranges and Zones 63
    The Importance of Calcium 65
    CALCIUMS AND FEEDING THE LIVER 66
RBTIOM Putting It All Together 68

RBTIOM Preface

RBTIOM is the acronym for the combination of **R**eams **B**iological **T**heory of **I**onization with the application of **O**riginal **M**edicine concepts and principles.

This book is designed to provide the basic concepts and principles of two complementary topics, i.e., Reams Biological Theory of Ionization (RBTI) and Original Medicine (OM), to empower the reader with a foundational understanding of how the combination can be used for achieving optimum health and vitality.

The reader will be exposed to the basics of the most powerful health system known to mankind, designed to prevent and reverse all chronic degenerative diseases. In addition, a very powerful scientifically based biochemical analysis, which can be run in less than ten minutes in your home, showcases the depth and breadth of the time-honored original medicine eight laws of health.

The objective is to present this complex mathematical tool in a user-friendly manner. A more detailed expansion of the RBTIOM concepts and principles will be provided in the book entitled <u>The Ultimate Answer to Health & Vitality: Reams Biological Theory of Ionization with Original Medicine.</u>

It is the clear intent of the author to meet the following objectives:

- Present the foundational Original Medicine and RBTI topics in a clear, coherent manner for both the general public and practitioners.
- Avoid the esoteric and complex underpinnings of the topics covered while maintaining the integrity of the information presented in terms of foundational Biblical and Dr. Carey A. Reams concepts and principles.
- Acknowledge the enormity and richness of the two topics while providing a solid foundation in the most important concepts and principles.
- Prayerfully distill my combined academic and practical experiences of over 30 years in the natural health field into a foundational understanding of God's time-honored natural laws of health with a powerful scientific, laboratory-level health evaluation and improvement tool that can be performed in the home and office environment.

May you continue to receive God's richest blessings as you carefully and prayerfully digest this material.

What is Original Medicine?

Original medicine draws its knowledge and inspiration from the Bible with its description of a Divine Creator, the origin of man, the original diet, and the original design for achieving perfect health and vitality. Honor and glory belong to God alone for all health since He is the Originator and Creator of all things. All human beings and their inventions, systems, power, and wisdom are subordinate to His power, wisdom, original design, and purpose.

Original medicine embraces the fact that God is the Author of the natural laws of health and has placed within our power the means for obtaining knowledge of these laws of health. Original medicine encourages putting forth the needed effort to obtain knowledge of God's laws of life and the simple means He has chosen to be employed for the achieving, maintaining, and restoration of health. It is our duty to preserve our physical and mental powers in the best possible condition so that we may effectively serve Him and our fellow man.

When sickness is the result of the transgression of natural law, we should seek to correct the error by prayerfully regaining harmony with both the moral and natural laws. Those who refuse to improve the light and knowledge that has been mercifully and lovingly placed within their reach are rejecting the beat means that God has provided them to promote spiritual as well as physical health and vitality.

The integrated and comprehensive use of God's eight laws of health make up the most powerful health-enhancing system known to man. These time-honored principles are the basis of the **original medicine** concept. As important as nutrition or a proper diet is in relation to good health, it can be quite meaningless in the absence of an integrated and comprehensive application of all the natural laws of health.

The effectiveness of all other methods of maintaining and enhancing health and vitality should be evaluated on the basis of their promotion of these foundational laws of health. We should be thankful for the power of these simple laws, apply them to ourselves, and then lovingly share them with our family, friends, and associates for a richer and healthier society, neighborhood, and world.

What is RBTI?

RBTI uses a mathematical formula to express the perfect health possible in the human biological system. The complex mathematical equation determines precisely where energy loss is occurring. The quick measurement of urine and saliva gives a remarkable view into how the entire body deals with food and fluid intake, digestion effectiveness, and excretion of wastes. Combined with gender, age, height, weight, and race, the equation looks at **energy in** and **energy out**, revealing energy gain or loss over time.

A move away from ideal numbers means indigestion, a loss or lack of energy, short circuits, and the beginning of depletion, deterioration, dysfunction, and destruction of healthy cells. When the numbers are close to the target, which is called "the healing zone," new cells are created in the body efficiently, making up all the different and unique tissues and organs of a perfectly healthy human – all naturally.

This measuring system describes how effectively and efficiently your body is creating **ENERGY**. If the numbers are away from perfect, the **CARBS** and **SALT** readings will either be **TOO HIGH** or **TOO LOW**. The pH of urine and saliva will either be **TOO FAST** or **TOO SLOW**. If your "numbers" don't match the equation, then you are losing energy, and it's this energy loss that causes the breakdown of the body, including tiredness, fatigue, health issues, aches, pains, injury, and slow recovery. The cause of this breakdown begins with mineral deficiency caused by an incorrect diet, incorrect hydration, lack of rest, lack of movement, and mental and emotional issues, just to name a few – all are contributing to energy loss.

This is **NOT** a system of Diagnosis; this is a system of Analysis. While medical tests diagnose and treat symptoms, this analysis looks at the cause of symptoms and corrects them at the true source of the cause.

The testing is a non-invasive process that reveals individual biochemical status after a urine and saliva analysis. It is a true post-digestion "insight." The results will indicate the best foods to eat, suggest what minerals will better serve the individual, and suggest what to do to reach an optimal level of health and well-being.

Simply, this is a system based on how the body separates matter and energy, uses that energy and then puts that energy back together again. Trillions of cells require enormous amounts of energy to rebuild and replace themselves. We need a balanced body biochemistry to increase and maintain our energy. The body is a miraculous healing machine. Through constant automatic adjustment, the body has an inbuilt **"tuning system."** The body will constantly look to balance biochemistry towards a **"perfect state"** for optimum health. The numbers used as the baseline is the reference point of perfect health.

A test is completed on the urine and saliva, and **"the numbers"** and interrelationships are then compared to the baseline. These results are used to create a nutritional program and lifestyle suggestions with the goal of encouraging the numbers into a **"healing zone"** or the ideal Range.

When one performs a test, their results are unique to them. The numbers are on a logarithmic scale with literally billions of combinations. Not one person is the same as the next; therefore, it is most unlikely that two individuals will have an identical wellness plan.

It is possible to predict an approaching disorder or health issue well before symptoms appear. The system is a true preventative disease tool, and by self-care, optimum health is achieved by correcting any required chemistry changes to the body before and during any illness. A lack of certain specific minerals usually makes it impossible for the body to maintain proper function and digest food effectively, therefore disabling the body's true digestion and healing potential.

We are looking at human health from the perspective of the cell. If the body is losing energy or is inefficient in digestion, then the body is in decline. Damage will continue to accumulate, which means symptoms will continue to worsen. Whether there is a health issue or a sports performance and recovery goal, this concept uses the same pathway back to optimum health. This is simply the process of ease or disease; energy continues to be lost, the body cannot heal efficiently, and damage accumulates. More specifically, cell damage accumulates. The progression toward disease, ill health, or lack of performance is caused by the depletion of minerals, resulting in a distortion of cells, disruption of biochemical signaling, and, eventually, the destruction of cells. With regular analysis and the client following suggestions, it doesn't take too long before there is an increase in energy and the quality of life is restored to an optimum level. Then, maintaining the numbers in the healing zone becomes a way of life.

This is a working explanation of the fundamental ionic energy composition and function of biological life. The loss of energy in all biological life is the beginning of disease. The purpose of an analysis is to identify previously unrecognized electro-biochemical dysfunctions taking place within the human body, thereby allowing the creation of a set of personal lifestyle recommendations that will address and reverse those unrecognized dysfunctional patterns. When correctly applied, the program offers the highest potential for perfect health.

To list a few of the benefits: greater energy, better sleep, higher sports performance, fast recovery, ease of movement in joints and muscles, weight gain or loss, balanced thinking, and emotional stability, just to name a few.

In essence, people become full of life!

What is RBTIOM?

RBTIOM is a combination of two systems for maximizing health potential and outcomes. It combines the most powerful system known to man for preventing and reversing all chronic degenerative diseases (**O**riginal **M**edicine) with the most powerful analytical tool known to man for identifying the major causes and contributors to compromised health outcomes (**RBTI**).

RBTI is the mathematical formula for perfect health. It identifies key deficiencies with a scientific analysis of organ and systemic energy loss that can be done in five minutes in your own home. As the numbers move away from perfect, there are a number of approaches that can be used to bring the numbers back to the healing and perfect zone. Of all the health protocols available, including both medical and alternative, the original medicine approach is the most effective and efficient way to achieve improved health and vitality.

There is no wisdom, and there is no knowledge that surpasses the wisdom and knowledge of God. He created us and provided all we need to sustain the optimal function of His creation on this side of heaven until we are reunited for eternity according to His **original** design for us **in His image and likeness**. Accordingly, no scientist or chemist can surpass God's ways and means.

The integrated and comprehensive application of God's eight laws of health, aka original medicine, according to individual requirements and capacities, as mathematically measured via RBTI, is the most powerful health system known to man. **Original Medicine** defines and actuates health. **RBTI** measures, analyzes, and manifests it in the mathematical analysis of urine and saliva.

The following summarizes the fundamental principles of RBTIOM:

- We are created by God in His image and likeness, and he has provided us with simple yet powerful health laws (**O**riginal **M**edicine) for sustaining His design and purpose for our health and vitality.
- Dr. Carey A. Reams, with his extensive scientific credentials, through prayer and fasting, discovered and promoted God's mathematical equation for perfect health (**RBTI**).
- RBTI showcases and validates the power of original medicine.
- RBTIOM sets the standard and is used to validate the effectiveness, or lack thereof, of other methods and approaches for improving health and vitality.

While acknowledging the complex mathematics and applied physics involved with RBTI, RBTIOM is an attempt by the author of this acronym to focus on empowerment as opposed to waxing eloquently on the complex underpinnings, many of which are beyond both the ability of both the author and the intended audiences.

THE PURPOSE OF RBTIOM IS NOT MAKE YOU AN EINSTEIN or DR. CAREY A. REAMS NO MORE THAN READING THE BIBLE WILL MAKE YOU A SAINT.

But just as rightful obedience to the Ten Commandments is the key to moral health and vitality, RBTIOM is an effort to offer our valued readers (both health enthusiasts and practitioners) a powerful system of original medicine, eight health laws, and a seven-number mathematical formula for experiencing perfect health and vitality – physically, mentally, emotionally, and spiritually.

The remainder of this book is designed to empower its readers with these RBTIOM concepts and principles.

$$PH = CS + 1.5 \quad \frac{6.4}{6.4} \quad 6.5C \quad .04m \quad \frac{3}{3}$$

PH = Perfect Health

CS = Common Sense

Perfect Health numbers are:

1.5 = % of Carbohydrates

6.4 = pH (for both urine and saliva)

6.5C = Conductivity or Salts (Electrical current reading)

.04M = Cellular Debris (in parts per million)

3 = Nitrate Nitrogen & Ammonia Nitrogen (Ureas)

Concepts of Original Medicine

(This is primarily an excerpt from the book Concepts of Original Medicine by Jim Sharps, N.D., H.D., Dr. N. Sc., Ph.D.)

THE EIGHT LAWS OF HEALTH

God made earth inhabitable for men and animals. All living things have been given the ability to use natural resources, such as the atmosphere (fresh air), the sun, water, etc. Our planet was designed to sustain life and, if used properly, provide good health and a comfortable living for every creature. God gave us natural laws so that we could lead well-balanced lives. Unfortunately, since leaving the Garden of Eden, mankind has been making his own laws regarding not only religion but also the care of his body.

God designed laws in this universe for everything that we do. The author of our moral laws is also the author of the natural laws. If we do not obey these laws, we must suffer the consequences! God gave us natural laws to live by. And if we want GOOD health, then we must put into practice all eight of these natural laws.

The Eight "Original Medicine" Laws of Health are:
1. Air
2. Water
3. Sunlight
4. Nutrition
5. Exercise
6. Rest
7. Temperance
8. Trust in Divine Power

Let's look at how these laws contribute to health and vitality in the following chapters.

PURE AIR IS ESSENTIAL FOR RADIANT HEALTH

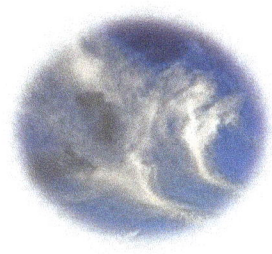

Air is the most important nutrient. This is obvious because as little as three minutes of deprivation will have very apparent and serious effects not only on our health but also on our very existence. In fact, Air provides 80% of the nutrients for our overall health and vitality.

Pure air is the first essential of a healthy body. We can live without food for several weeks and water for several days, but we cannot live without air. Air is so important and necessary that we cannot even commit suicide by just stopping breathing. If we hold our breath to the point of blacking out, our brainstem automatically takes over and causes us to start breathing again.

One of the important functions of air is to provide oxygen for the combustion (metabolism) of ingested nutrients. Without adequate oxygen, each cell cannot complete its functions. Without adequate oxygen, the cells and organs that eliminate the waste products of metabolism cannot function effectively. When the supply of oxygen is diminished, waste and poisons can accumulate. Any health treatment that does not encourage the use of good, clean, and fresh air will be significantly compromised in its effectiveness.

Pure, natural air is a gift from God. The rays of the sun sterilize it. Rainwater washes and cleanses it. It is purified by the synergistic action of plant life. Plants use our exhaled carbon dioxide and, in exchange, provide us with fresh supplies of life-giving oxygen. With the disappearance of many of our forests and the effects of industrially generated pollutants, the supply of fresh, pure air is almost nonexistent in our day-to-day living and working environments. Instead of life-giving oxygen in abundance, there is an abundance of carbon dioxide, carbon monoxide, and other pollutants from tobacco smoke, automobile emissions, industrial wastes, burning vegetation, etc.

Pure, fresh air oxygenates and enlivens the body. Impure air is one of the greatest causes of poor health. Health-conscious people should be knowledgeable about their environments and the quality of the air they breathe. Air quality tends to be best in the early morning and late evening. The best supply of clean, fresh air can be found in the mountains, in large wooded areas, near large bodies of water, and in some remote places far from industry and automobiles.

Clean, fresh air is negatively charged, and polluted air is positively charged. In instances where indoor air is poor, a negative ion generator can be used to improve air quality. There is no real substitute, however, for fresh, clean outdoor air. Because fresh air is so important to health, we need to make an effort to breathe natural, clean air, for example, during outdoor morning exercise. This will impart to us a vitality that is superior and cannot be matched by breathing stale, re-circulated air or that found in smoky rooms, congested offices, or noisy factories.

The effects of poor air quality are well known. Cigarette smoking is linked to emphysema and lung cancer; even second-hand smoke is linked to sudden infant death syndrome (SIDS) in babies. Discomfort and symptoms related to office environments have led to such phrases as sick-building syndrome. This is particularly noted in sealed buildings with centrally controlled mechanical ventilation. Associated conditions include allergies, infections, Legionnaire's disease, and worsening of asthma because of air-borne irritants.

Some Important Qualities of Air

1. Air is a food. In fact, it is more essential than any other food and must be present to perform many vital functions. The oxygen in the air is carried by the blood to every cell in the body and is essential for cellular metabolism.
2. Air contains electricity. Fresh air charges your nerves and muscles with electricity and increases your energy.
3. Air is a healing agent. A wound will not heal without air. It acts as both a purifier and a deodorizer.
4. Fresh air acts as an agent in producing a more positive mental attitude. It strengthens and nourishes the nervous system. Foul air is depressing and stressful to your body.
5. The oxygen in the air is replenished by the leaves of trees. We, in turn, breathe out carbon dioxide, an essential nutrient for plants! God created this synergistic cycle so that we would always have fresh supplies of oxygen to maintain optimum health.

Daily exposure to fresh air is very important for vibrant health. Each day, you should begin with an air bath. Exposing your body to the air with as little clothing as is practical can be very refreshing and revitalizing for your entire body.

Basic deep breathing can be incorporated into your daily routine. All bodily functions, including proper digestion, need clean air, and proper breathing aids assimilation and metabolism. Most people tend to breathe significantly less than their true capacity. Deep breathing starts in the diaphragm and is extremely important to physical health.

The lung is a major organ of elimination. Shallow breathing limits the amount of carbon dioxide and other harmful gases that can be eliminated through your lungs. Breathing should be relaxed and done within your capacity. Breathing in (inhalation) energizes the body, and breathing out (exhalation) relaxes the body. When using breathing exercises, it is important that your exhalation be at least as long as your inhalation and most authorities recommend that exhalation be slightly longer than inhalation.

Most aerobic activities encourage deep breathing to promote the functional integrity of the respiratory system. Certain disciplines like yoga, martial arts, and several holistic techniques encourage deep, controlled, and health-promoting breathing.

In summary, breathing is the simplest and most important bodily function for sustaining our bodies. Deep breathing, exercise that promotes breathing, and breathing fresh, pure air are all ways to provide the oxygen that our bodies need and promote radiant health.

PURE WATER IS ESSENTIAL FOR RADIANT HEALTH

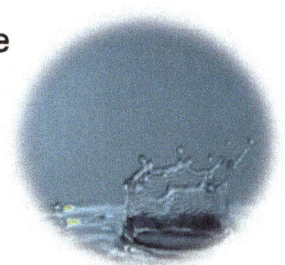

The most precious of all liquids is water. We can live without water for perhaps a week or two at the most, and deficiencies in this area are very well understood and documented.
Interestingly, our earth is 70 to 75% water, and our bodies are also 70 to 75% water, demonstrating the model of abundance and availability: what man needed most is what God created in abundance.

"The planet is 70-75% water, and so are our bodies—we are an exact template of the planet."

The body of a 150-pound man contains approximately 105 pounds of water. Water is essential for the function of every cell of the body. Almost every cell and tissue of our body not only contains water and is continually bathed in fluid but also requires water to perform its functions! The gray matter of the brain is approximately 85 percent water, the blood is approximately 83 percent water, and the muscles are approximately 75 percent water. All major processes in the body, including circulation, digestion, and elimination, require the presence of water. Body temperature is regulated by the evaporation of water from the skin. Because water is so essential to every cell and every function of the body, the kidneys reabsorb and recycle water as much water as possible. However, significant amounts of water are continuously being excreted to carry waste products in the urine, so the body's supply of water must be constantly replenished.

Health-conscious people should be knowledgeable about their environment and the quality of the water they use. Water pollution abounds because of contamination by sewage pumped into rivers and oceans; runoff from garbage dumps; oil spills; industrial wastes such as mercury, lead, and polychlorinated biphenols (PCBs); chemical fertilizers and pesticide residues; and so forth. Many of these substances are present in public drinking water because the law allows "acceptable levels." Mandated chlorination of public water adds yet another chemical. Natural, pure water is the best source of water. Still, for those who only have access to tap water, water filtration systems or bottled water are often the most practical means of getting optimum water quality. For most purposes, especially for cleansing and fasting programs, distilled water provides the best results.

Water is imperative to maintaining or regaining health. It is important to ensure adequate water intake to maintain bodily functions. A lack of the sensation of thirst is not always the best indicator of the body's need for water; some people do not feel thirsty until their bodies are quite dehydrated.

Your body requires approximately 64 to 80 ounces of water (8 to 10 eight-ounce glasses) a day. A general rule is one ounce of water for every two pounds of body weight, modified to meet special circumstances such as activity level, outside temperature, and health status. This recommendation of 8 to 10 glasses a day is for a cooked-food-oriented diet. However, living a natural lifestyle and eating a natural diet consisting primarily of fruits and vegetables provides the body with a built-in supply of water. Since fruits and vegetables are high water-content foods (more than 70 percent water), less additional drinking water is required. Most animals in the wild live on fruits and vegetables and drink very modest amounts of water. In addition, the water contained in fruits and vegetables has been distilled by the synergistic action of the sun and provides pure, clean, thirst-quenching, and life-giving water. Eating an adequate amount of live, fresh fruits and vegetables gives the body an abundance of the purest naturally distilled water, full of fragrance, organic minerals, and life-giving nutrients.

Altering the water content of foods by excessive cooking and processing compromises the quality of the food and its water content. When unnatural, processed foods are taken into the body, nature tries to counteract them by diluting them. This, in turn, causes thirst. Satisfying this thirst with the introduction of large quantities of unnatural fluids can be very distressful and harmful to the optimum performance of our bodies. Over-consumption of fluid, even water, causes several problems, including bloating, excessive water retention, distention of blood vessels and organs, and other harmful results. It can also overtax the kidneys and cause excessive urination.

When required, water is best taken between meals and should be sipped, not gulped down. It should be at room temperature or warmed for best results. Iced water, in particular, can be very harmful to the internal organs, especially the kidneys. It tends to shock and put the internal organs into spasm. Digestion is stopped until the water can be warmed to body temperature, thereby delaying or causing incomplete food breakdown.

Water is also beneficial externally. It can be used to reduce the heat of the body in cases of fever, increase the heat of the body in cases of low vitality, cleanse the skin, and tonify the body.

Hydrotherapy, properly administered colonics, contrast foot baths, showers, and steam baths are some of the external uses of water that promote and maintain health. Hydrotherapy is a special therapy that uses the application of hot and cold water treatments. Colon hydrotherapy uses warm water to gently clean out and stimulate reflex points in the colon. Contrast showers and foot baths, which employ alternating hot and cold water, relax the muscles, improve circulation, and strengthen the immune system. Steam baths open and cleanse the pores of the skin.

In summary, water is one of the simplest and most important substances we can use for sustaining our bodies. Water taken internally, particularly in the purified form found in fruits and vegetables, and water administered externally are ways in which we can care for our bodies and promote radiant health.

SUNLIGHT IS ESSENTIAL FOR RADIANT HEALTH

We can live without sunlight for extended periods of time, longer than without both air and water, but not without serious consequences. All life on earth depends on the energy of the sun. In short, all life on earth, including human beings, would cease to exist if there was no sunshine.

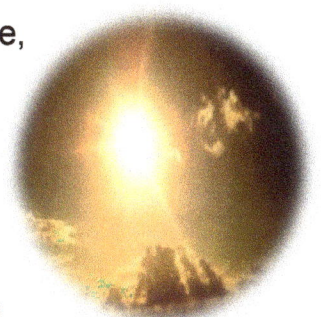

Sunshine helps maintain the ambient temperatures of the earth. In this way, it supports plant and animal existence and is a vital ingredient in our environment.

Sunlight is composed of many different energy levels transmitted through electromagnetic waves. The rays of the sun expose the body to three types of light of different wavelengths:

1. Invisible light. The invisible light generated by the sun includes both ultraviolet and infrared light. Ultraviolet light (5 percent of solar radiation) provides the majority of the biological effects, both positive and negative, to the body. Infrared light (54 percent of solar emissions) provides warmth.

2. Visible light (40 percent of the solar radiation)

3. Other types of waves: shorter cosmic rays, gamma rays, and x-rays; longer radio waves and electromagnetic waves.

Some obvious benefits of the sun are the production of vitamin D in the skin, improved vitamin and mineral absorption, particularly calcium, and overall improvement in metabolic function and efficiency. In addition to the known nutrient-giving properties of the sun, there are many complex and even unknown benefits. As a secondary benefit, the abundant energy and life-giving properties that sunlight gives to the plant kingdom have similar positive effects on humans who eat those plants.

Daily sunlight is required for all healthy, living things in order to develop, grow, and flourish. As little as 20 minutes of exposure to sunlight a day has powerful positive effects on your body. The full-spectrum light and energy provided by the sun supplies the subtle, vibratory energy underlying all plant and human function. Exposure to the sun results in a healthy-looking complexion, energized blood, and overall good health.

Some of the important effects of the sun on your body are as follows:

1. Chemical. It unlocks the vitamins in your food. The process of digestion is incomplete without sunshine. The more light and heat we receive from the sun, the less heavy food we require. Sunlight, in effect, controls the chemistry of the blood.
2. Physical. Sunlight warms your body and, at the same time, energizes it. Sunshine helps and encourages every important function of the body. When the sun shines on your skin, it quickly stores up a tremendous amount of energy in your body. The nerve endings absorb the vibrant energy and transmit this energy to your entire nervous system. Natural sunlight contains the full spectrum of colors, which provides the best medium for visual acuity. The underlying energy systems of your body are constantly feeding on and storing up the life-giving elements from the sun's rays. Sunshine, like air, acts as a stimulant, tonic, and healer. Some bacteria cannot live in direct sunlight, and many diseases are curable by allowing the sun to come in direct contact with the diseased part of the body for various periods of time. Sunshine is both a natural and effective healing agent. Eating in sunlight, when practical, enhances digestion and encourages a natural diet. A healthy, natural diet, in turn, enhances interest in and tolerance of sunlight. If your body has the right nutrients, it will respond very favorably to sunlight.
3. Psychological. Exposure to sunshine offers the experience of peace, joy, happiness, and a feeling of relief and freedom. The mind immediately senses that the body is in its natural medium, and the thoughts begin to take on a more lofty aspect.

In modern times, we noticed a decline in the interest in sunshine. Until a few years ago, the general public practically ignored the marvelous health-giving power of sunlight, and was familiar to only a handful of people. Now, there seems to be an awakening to the wonderful beneficial effects of the sun's rays on the health and vitality of the human body and the ill effects caused by a lack of sunlight. Insufficient sunlight results in a pale complexion lowered physical vitality, and poor health.

Psychologically, it has been linked to seasonal affective disorder (SAD), a mood disorder of depression that appears during the winter months when there is less sunlight. On the other hand, overexposure to sunlight should be avoided at all times, especially exposure to midday sun in the summer months. As in many areas of life, the dictum "Moderation in those things that are healthful and abstinence from all things that are harmful" applies to sunlight.

In summary, sunlight is one of the simplest and most important substances we can use for sustaining our bodies. Sunshine is free, and its rays invigorate the body in many ways that promote radiant health.

NUTRITION IS ESSENTIAL FOR RADIANT HEALTH

God made our bodies and our minds. Then He turned the responsibility of their maintenance, along with a set of health laws, over to us, to our keeping. If we eat the foods God intended us to use in the way God intended us to use them, then we will have good, strong, healthy bodies. If we don't follow these dietary rules, then our bodies will suffer as a result and eventually become diseased.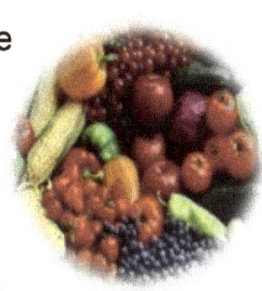

Fundamentally, the best foods for physical nourishment and health are living, whole foods as they were created by God and provided by nature. All the knowledge we have gained since the beginning of time continually supports this simple fact. Nature, in the form of plant foods, supplies all the food and medicine we need for physical health. Nature provides the most perfect food laboratory that yields an abundant menu of wholesome vitamins, minerals, proteins, carbohydrates, fats, and other essential known and unknown nutrients. Fruits, vegetables, nuts, grains, seeds, and edible herbs, properly prepared and in adequate amounts, supply all the nutrients required for developing and maintaining optimum health. Especially when eaten raw, the life of the food in the form of enzymes is still present and is highly beneficial to the body. This forms the basis of the dietary principles of original medicine.

In my book, Basic Principles of Total Health, I present a "hierarchy of nutrients" that ranks types of foods--from the best to the worst--as far as their ability to promote optimum, radiant health. This hierarchy is an alternative to the popular food pyramid, and it provides a perspective on nutrition that is in harmony with the original medicine concepts and principles.

The meaning of proper diet goes beyond eating a variety of healthy foods. It also includes eating those foods in the proper quantities and at the right time of the day. At one time, people grew and ate their own (native) simple foods, depending upon where they lived. Today, the world has become so small due to communication and rapid transportation that we now have food on our tables from around the world whenever we choose. In the sheer abundance of available foods, we have greater temptations today and greater opportunities to overeat.

Indulgence of appetite and gluttony are prevalent and are ruinous to good health. Alcoholic and stimulating drinks consumed as companions to poor food choices further compromise our health. The right quantity of food and the correct time of day are both extremely important in maintaining good health. The breakfast meal should be the most nourishing meal of the day because it supplies the nutrients to carry us through the day. Instead, sugar-rich foods and coffee is consumed as a breakfast. This causes a quick rise in blood sugar and then a later fall in blood sugar with a sudden hunger that prompts overeating.

Not only do we have inadequate eating habits, but we also snack and eat continually throughout the day and evening, forcing our stomachs to work constantly digesting food hour after hour. The evening meal should be light so that the stomach is empty before retiring in the evening. Instead, in the evening, we eat large complex meals and extra helpings of dessert. This causes our digestive system to work all night digesting the food. Like the body, the stomach, too, needs rest. Without rest, it becomes prone to disease.

But even with worldwide shipping and the availability of many new natural foods, we have ignored this source of health and continue to turn to manufactured foods that are high in sugar, high in fat, and low in nutrition. Instead of putting fruits, vegetables, nuts, grains, seeds, and edible herbs on our tables and enjoying these whole foods with their full complement of nutrients and healthful benefits, we prefer to eat white bread, white sugar, saturated fats, and commercially prepared foods that have been stripped of many nutrients only to be artificially "enriched" with a few vitamins and minerals. In America, we have a whole new generation that has been brought up on junk-food meals consisting of hamburgers, colas, candy bars, fried foods, etc. This diet has not only formed bad nutritional habits, but it has taken away a liking and a taste for the natural foods that are essential to the growth and health of the body. Consequently, we are experiencing a prevalent increase in diseases, even among the very young. Pediatricians note an outbreak of diseases previously seen only in adults--diabetes, obesity, and, more recently, kidney stones—all attributable to a poor diet in young people. Malnourished mothers eating nutritionally poor diets produce babies with even more compromised health. With the diseased conditions present in the animal kingdom, eating a flesh diet affects our physical, mental, emotional, and moral lives. It is almost impossible to live a patient, pure, healthful life while ingesting diseased animal products. These modern and yet impoverished eating habits have taken their toll on whole nations, and combating diseases caused by poor nutrition is now a way of life.

In summary, nutrition is an incredibly important factor in maintaining good health. Fruits, vegetables, grains, nuts, and herbs as whole foods are the most healthful. Commercially prepared foods have far fewer nutrients, and we compound this lack of nutrients by eating too much of the wrong foods at the wrong time. Unlike fresh air, fresh water, and sunshine, wholesome foods are not free. Still, God has given us the opportunity and the responsibility of using knowledge to make healthy food choices that invigorate the body and promote radiant health.

EXERCISE IS ESSENTIAL FOR RADIANT HEALTH

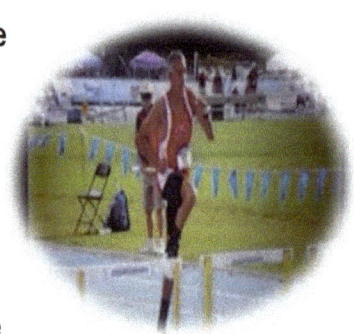

Exercise is another law for the optimal performance of your body. It contributes to both the nourishment of your body and the elimination of waste. The fundamental principle of exercise as it relates to health is movement. Without movement, all life ceases to exist. In death, all systems of your body--including the heart, brain, and circulatory system--stop "moving." If anything in the universe stops moving, its function is altered.

This underlying principle of movement is the factor that promotes and supports optimal health. Movement engages all the major systems in your body, including the muscular, skeletal, nervous, endocrine (glands), and lymphatic systems.

In general, most people use only about 50 of the more than 600 muscles in their bodies. This often results in the overuse of less than 10 percent of our muscles with relatively inactivity of the rest, which can result in several disease processes. Using a variety of individualized exercises or movements (based on genetic or environmental conditions) offers many advantages to optimizing health and wellness.

Anything that encourages the natural movement of the body contributes to health. The type and amount of exercise you choose are subject to the same rules of temperance and balance as the foods you eat. Whether walking, running, swimming, doing aerobics, yoga, tai chi, martial arts, weightlifting, gardening, or pursuing any other activity, the following principles contribute to a healthy approach to exercise.

Exercise should:
- be enjoyable and relaxing
- be free of strain and pain
- use as many muscles and joints as is feasible
- use a variety of movements
- balance strength with flexibility and stretching
- help you to breathe more deeply

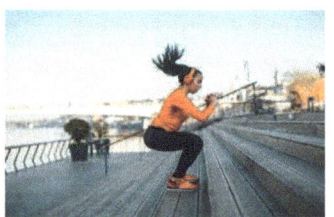

Some Important Benefits of Exercise

Regular exercise is not only a preventive measure; it also works to maintain health at its best. There are many benefits of physical exercise. Some of them include the following.

- Exercise makes one more energetic and gives a sense of well-being.
- Exercise helps to lower high blood pressure. The New England Journal of Medicine published a study that found that aerobic exercise significantly lowered blood pressure in patients with hypertension.
- Exercise strengthens bones. Research conducted at Washington University School of Medicine in St. Louis demonstrated that a woman can increase her bone mass by 2 to 3 percent per year (for as long as the study was conducted) by weight-bearing exercises.
- Exercise promotes an increase in HDL cholesterol (good cholesterol). A study of nearly 3,000 men revealed that exercise was associated with higher HDL levels.
- Exercise helps in the management of diabetes. Harvard researchers documented that exercise decreases the risk of developing diabetes in adulthood. Exercise increases the ability of cell membranes to transport glucose into muscle cells. This particular transportation is not dependent on insulin, thus lowering the insulin requirement.
- Exercise improves brain oxygen availability and circulation in those with Alzheimer's disease. In a study examining the communication skills of two groups of Alzheimer's patients, more than 40 percent of the group in a walking exercise program experienced significant improvement in communication skills, whereas the group who were given conversation lessons experienced no significant improvement.
- Exercise improves mental health. A study of patients not suffering from Alzheimer's disease showed measurable improvement in memory after an aerobic exercise program of nine to ten weeks. With increased activity, older persons showed improved mental function. There was a clear linear relationship between the level of activity and the level of mental ability. Through regular, active use of the body, one can discover a greater sense of well-being, far greater vitality, and a calmer, more relaxed attitude toward daily pressures.
- Exercise improves cardiac function. It strengthens the heart, making it more efficient so that it is able to pump a greater volume of blood with each contraction.

- Exercise improves the quality of life. A consensus panel convened by the National Institute of Health identified other important benefits in quality of life from exercise, such as better mental health, decreased stress, decreased anxiety and depression, and decreased risk of certain cancers.

In 1998, the Oregonian published a story about an elderly man, Ben Levinson, 103 years old, to be precise, who set a world record for the shot-put for men over 100. He threw the ball 10 feet and 1.25 inches. But for Ben, the achievement was to be throwing at all, at over 100 years! Thirteen years before, Ben Levinson was a depressed, unfit 90-year-old, shuffling around, frail, and ready for the grave. Ben had become dependent and weak through a lack of exercise. Fortunately for Ben, he met Dave Crawley, an athletics trainer, who challenged him to feel 80 again. Ben began a training program, walking 20 minutes a day at 2.5 miles per hour and weight-training three or four times a week. "He's grown 2 inches just with better posture and more confidence," says Crawley.

If a fitness program could do that for this 90-year-old, just think what it could do for you.

In summary, exercise is an incredibly important factor in maintaining good health. The wonderful thing about exercise is that you can begin reaping its rewards regardless of how old you are when you begin. Again, God has given us the opportunity and the responsibility of using knowledge to make healthful choices that invigorate the body and promote radiant health.

Adequate Rest is Essential for Radiant Health

Adequate rest is imperative for optimum health. Rest brings restoration and replenishes the resources we use. Without rest, the body's process of catabolism (breaking down) overrides that of anabolism (building up), resulting in disease and compromised health.

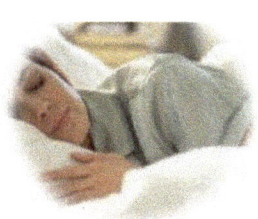

Sleep is the most important medium for rest. Short naps, peaceful and relaxing environments, mental quietness, and the avoidance of stress also contribute to rest for your body.

Given the fact that, in one day, the heart beats over 100,000 times, pumping blood through miles of blood vessels, we speak thousands of words, breathe 23,000 times, move major muscles hundreds of times, and operate some 15 to 20 billion brain cells, no wonder sleep is important in restoring our energy and maintaining health. As Shakespeare wrote: "Sleep wraps up the raveled sleeve of care."

A newborn sleeps an average of 20 hours a day, a 6-year-old sleeps about 10 hours, a 12-year-old sleeps about 9 hours, and an adult sleeps approximately 8 hours. Whether these averages are optimal varies, depending upon the individual. Breslow and Belloc, in their famous Alameda County study, showed that persons obtaining 8 to 9 hours of sleep per night seemed to have better health outcomes than those sleeping shorter or longer periods of time.

Occasionally, there are individuals, such as Ben Franklin and Thomas Edison, who can get by with 4 or 5 hours of sleep a night, but these individuals are the exceptions rather than the rule. Many who only sleep for short periods of time at night also take short catnaps throughout the day. Albert Einstein required at least 9 hours of sleep. Adequate sleep should prevent sleepiness and drowsiness during the day and promote a sense of well-being and alertness.

Students who study all night prior to an examination often suffer the consequences of sleep deprivation manifested in inferior grades. Work schedules that do not permit adequate sleep may result in increased inattention in the workplace and accidents and errors.

According to sleep experts, we go through various stages and certain sleep cycles. Each cycle lasts approximately 90 minutes. We start with stage one sleep, the lightest stage, and then progress to a deeper stage two sleep. Stage three sleep is related to delta-wave brain activity, which is the slowest and most relaxed brain wave activity. Stage four is our deepest stage of sleep. The most powerful healing and rebuilding take place during the fourth stage of sleep, which lasts approximately 20 to 45 minutes. Then, we gradually return through stage three, stage two, and stage one sleep. A complete and uninterrupted cycling through these stages allows us to awaken refreshed without an alarm clock, and this significantly contributes to optimal health.

In cases of compromised health or excessive physical and mental activity, rest is imperative for restoring and supporting your body's natural healing ability. It is the most important factor for replenishing spent resources.

Sleep patterns also influence the secretion of the following hormones:
1. Cortisol. This hormone is secreted during the second half of the sleep period. It prepares the body for the activity of the next day. Cortisol has numerous effects, influencing blood glucose levels, regulating sodium and potassium concentrations, regulating blood pressure, and influencing muscle strength. One of its most important actions is its anti-inflammatory effect. Regular sleep habits result in regular patterns of cortisol secretion.
2. Growth hormone. This hormone is secreted at its maximal rate during sleep. Its hormone affects glucose and amino acid metabolism.
3. Melatonin. Secretion rates increase during the night but may have more of a role to play in sexual regulation than anything to do with sleep regulation.

There are a number of other factors that can have a positive or negative influence on sleep. These include the following.

- Regular exercise and the avoidance of excessive fatigue during the day are conducive to good sleep at night.

- The last meal of the day should be a light one taken a few hours prior to retiring. However, it should be skipped or consist of something light, like fruit, if sufficient time is not available for the stomach to digest the food before retiring.

- The stomach should not be full before going to sleep, as the stomach needs to be resting along with other parts of the body. The digestive system tends to use more energy than any other major system of the body, including the circulatory, respiratory, and nervous system.

Therapeutic fasting provides another energy-conserving and resting opportunity for your body.

- Avoidance of alcohol, tobacco, caffeine, and other chemical substances that interfere with normal sleep patterns is advised.
- The time preceding retirement should be free of arguments, exciting TV, and stressful events. It should be a quiet time to wind down the day's activity and prepare for rest.
- A warm, not hot, bath may help relaxation before bed. Use the many relaxation techniques, including massage, meditation, and prayer, to provide valuable rest that contributes to health and wellness. In addition to natural sleep and a temperate diet and lifestyle, relaxation techniques contribute to vibrant energy and optimum health.
- Irregularity in rising and going to bed, shift work, travel across time zones, and weekend changes in sleep all militate against good sleep patterns.
- A quiet bedroom, free of bright light and noise, properly ventilated, and of a comfortable temperature aids in sleeping.
- Medical conditions such as sleep apnea, respiratory disorders, cardiac conditions, phobias, and other psychiatric disorders may require professional assistance.

When God created the earth, He created night as a period of daily rest for both man and animals. The Lord our Creator knows that our bodies need a balanced daily rest-- physically, mentally, emotionally, and socially. At the close of the creation week, God Himself "rested" on the seventh day as an example to man of how to rest from his labors each week because He also knows that to function optimally, we also need a weekly rest. Not only did God "rest' but He also blessed this day. "Remember the Sabbath day, to keep it holy. Six days you shall labor and do all your work: but the seventh day is the Sabbath of the Lord your God: in it, you shall do no work: you, nor your son, nor your daughter, nor your manservant, nor your maidservant, nor your cattle, nor your stranger who is within your gates." (Exodus 20:8-10)

Rest at the appropriate times is beneficial and contains a blessing. The Bible says that there should be daily rest as well as a weekly rest, and even modern man has found that just such a rest meets all his needs by providing a much-needed break from the demands of the work. In addition, the Sabbath provides a special blessing not only of rest but also of fellowship. The Lord wants us to have fellowship with Him, especially on the Sabbath day, for He created us as His children. Part of the blessing of the Sabbath rest comes as we support and relate to each other. Service to others provides a powerful rest from the self-focused and egocentric activities that often encumber us. The Sabbath was made for man, not man for the Sabbath! Regular sleep and weekly rest empowers us to be receptive to the blessing of God so that He can fill our lives with His many blessings!

Even during periods of greatest stress and activity with deadlines, rest is essential. During World War II, increased productivity was achieved, not by a continuous, non-stop work schedule to increase production that was first tried, but later by a 48-hour workweek. This demonstrated that, even under the pressures of war, people have limitations on their work capabilities and must rest if they are to do their best. On July 29, 1941, six months before the entry of the United States into the war, Prime Minister Winston Churchill announced in the House of Commons, "If we are to win this war, it will be by staying power. For this reason, we must have one holiday per week and one week holiday per year." And this was voted into law!

Periodic rests include annual vacations. These vacations are not necessarily periods of inactivity but of engagement in activities normally outside the scope of the daily routine. These times provide mental and emotional restitution, help stimulate creativity, and strengthen family relationships.

In summary, rest is an incredibly important factor in maintaining good health. The wonderful thing about rest is God has provided times of rest throughout the week—nightly rest for sleep and a weekly Sabbath rest to fellowship with him and rest from our labors. Again, God has given us the opportunity and the responsibility of using knowledge to make healthful choices to rest the body and promote radiant health.

Temperance is Essential for Radiant Health

Temperance means to be moderate or sparing, using self-restraint and self-control. So, when we speak of temperance, we are speaking of balance and self-control. It is the underlying factor of balance and rhythm of all the other laws of health, i.e., not too much and not too little, but just right for overall balance and integration of the laws of health for optimum health and vitality.

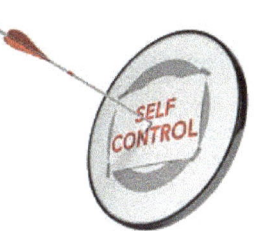

Temperance and self-control are necessary to avoid health-destroying behaviors. Is there any sense in the moderate use of arsenic or strychnine? Definitely not! Everyone knows these are deadly poisons. However, some things, even things commonly used by many people—things like tobacco, alcohol, and addictive substances—are best totally avoided because of their poisonous effect on the body. However, alcohol, tobacco, and other drugs are enticing because they are promoted as fun, stimulating, and as a release from stress and pain. Even many innocent-appearing popular beverages contain drugs.

Theophylline lurks in tea, and caffeine is hidden in most coffee and colas. Fruit-flavored wine coolers contain alcohol. Using alcohol, tobacco, and other drugs in any amount is hazardous because they often lead to addiction and harm. Even some prescription drugs can be addictive, and they must be used with great caution and only when necessary. Drugs destroy the purity of the mind when they cause addiction; drugs destroy the purity of the soul when intoxication leads to abuse, inappropriate sex, or violent behavior. Drugs destroy the purity of the body when they cause disease and even death. Instead of artificial stimulants with a subsequent crash, get your highs from exercise and enjoying the beauty of God's created world. In place of chemical depressants and stimulants, get your relaxation from sunlight, water, and rest.

Temperance, moderation, and balance are principles that underlie all other health factors. Although moderation is usually associated with avoiding harmful things like processed foods, caffeine, nicotine, alcohol, drugs, and other waste elements, it also includes the wise and judicious use of good things.

Overeating and poor combinations of good food, over-supplementation with vitamins, indiscriminate use of herbs and other specialized products, and unbalanced amounts of exercise and rest can compromise optimum physical health. Moderation means using good common sense guided by the laws of health in God's word, the Bible. Moderation in the diet is rewarded with mental and moral vigor. If moderation is not part of our everyday life, it is easier to succumb to the temptation of things that injure our health. Moderation provides the balance and self-control that permit the highest attainment of our physical, mental, and spiritual development.

In summary, temperance is an incredibly important factor in maintaining good health. Temperance means to abstain from everything harmful and to use judiciously that which is beneficial. Again, God has given us the opportunity and the responsibility of using knowledge to be temperate and make healthful choices that promote radiant health.

TRUST IN DIVINE POWER IS ESSENTIAL FOR RADIANT HEALTH

Of all the eight laws of natural health, this law should be the most sacredly cherished because our every breath, good health, and the essence of all healing come from the Creator and Sustainer of all the laws of health and vitality.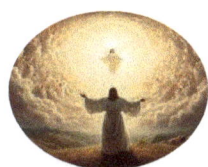

All great civilizations have been founded on religious beliefs and moral values that lead to an orderly society. Belief in spiritual values is a strong motivator to treat others well and to develop peaceful human relationships. History demonstrates that faithless and amoral societies become so corrupt they cannot survive. Belief is characteristic of science as well as religion. Just as faith in a scientific principle is verified when tests produce consistent results, faith in God is validated when it brings consistent and satisfying results. Studies indicate that those with regular spiritual practices who meet with a faith community live longer, live better, and are far less likely to have a stroke or heart attack. Faith can empower you to overcome stress and destructive habits. Belief can give you peace of mind and enable you to reach your full potential through positive choices.

All of God's creation relies on God completely. The planets and their suns orbit in an orderly fashion through space, rotating at enormous speeds on their axis while racing along their lines of travel. The animals hunt for their food, but it is God's hand that sends them their fare. "Consider the ravens, for they neither sow nor reap...yet God feeds them" (Luke 12:24). Even the flowers are under His care. "Consider the lilies, see how they grow; they neither toil nor spin, but even Solomon in all his glory could not clothe himself like one of these." (Luke 12:27) It is the human race alone that does not always recognize its total dependence on God's goodness and blessings. The God who made the world and all things in it, since He is Lord of heaven and earth...He Himself gives to all life and breath to all things...though He is not far from each one of us for in Him we live and move and have our being" (Acts 17:24-28).

Everyone needs to believe in something eternal and stable for viability and long-term health. Health at the spiritual level synergistically produces health at all levels in the mind and body. Your mind is energized with the vibrant health of positive thinking and emotions. Your body is ruled by the mind, and the body works to achieve Divine sustenance, not just subsistence.

Challenges that we face at the physical or mental level can compromise our ability to focus on our spiritual growth and development. Like air, which is abundantly supplied and easily available, the spiritual element of our being is easy to take for granted and overlook, even though it so pervasively and abundantly provides for our life and well-being.

Spiritual realization is available to all who are seeking wisdom and truth. Many squander this powerful and abundantly provided path to total health, but the few who truly set aside some quiet time to embrace the perfect and mysterious aspect of the spirit will find it. "Ask, and it will be given to you, seek and you will find, knock at the door and it will be opened to you." (Matthew 7:7-9) When you hear the prompting of your spirit.

(God's voice speaking to you quietly), listen, and you will be rewarded with renewed health and wellness.

A spiritual life is available to all of us, regardless of our station in life or level of performance. This is the one aspect of our being where we are all on a level playing field. It is the most powerful force of our being. An ounce of spiritual health can transcend pounds of physical and mental problems. Many mysterious and miraculous cures testify to this truly awesome phenomenon. Those wise enough to accept and capitalize on this aspect of their being can create the physiological and mental nutrients to overcome obstacles to achieving optimal health.

Spiritual growth and nourishment is a major aspect of all religions or philosophies. There are many paths that mankind has experienced during the quest for spiritual realization. Many sincere and well-intentioned religious organizations try to claim sole ownership of this realm. Still, the wisdom of men and institutions will always fall short of the enormous wisdom and power of the Creator of men.

Relying solely on human knowledge, science, and its institutions will always compromise total health at all levels of our being, especially at the spiritual level. The mysteries still to be unraveled far outweigh the knowledge we have gained during our brief history here on Earth. Spiritual health that is pure, peaceful, loving, and sincere is available to each of us.

While the spiritual part of our being is the most powerful aspect of human existence, it also tends to be both extremely complex and underutilized by many, and yet simply and powerfully utilized by some. What causes us to fall short of maximizing our spiritual support and nourishment? Don't we all want total health and happiness in our lives? The questions are easy, but the answers are not as simple. There are many distractions, including the daily activities of earning a livelihood, our natural pleasure-seeking ways, etc. At another level, our pride, selfish motives, arrogant sense of self-worth, and refusal to accept the truth can also be stressful burdens that must be eliminated before we can experience true spiritual health.

Once we understand and appreciate our relative insignificance from a universal perspective and humbly submit to and accept the spiritual prompting of God as given to us through a pure and healthy mind, we begin the process of waste elimination that will eventually lead to spiritual growth. Regardless of age, wealth, or wisdom, we are relatively powerless until we center our spiritual growth on an eternal God.

Spiritual health keeps our entire being in balance. It provides healthy soil that brings forth good fruit. It prevents us from being overweight and overbearing.

Just as fruits and vegetables are the staples for supporting our physical health, unconditional love and forgiveness are the primary staples for supporting spiritual health. Peace, joy, humility, and wisdom are the nuts, seeds, grains, and legumes that round out a complete whole food diet that supports our spiritual health.

As we develop a relationship with our Creator, we experience a new and improved body, mind, and spirit. As we selflessly share our newfound pearls of health and vitality with our neighbors, we improve our health, as well as that of our neighbors and our planet. The power of love, which is the life force of our spirit, creates, as it were, a new life and a new earth for us. Trusting in the Divine power that created us enables the harmonious integration of body, mind, and spirit. The earthly goal of physical health, which is temporal, is transcended to include spiritual health, which is eternal.

The following are health-promoting items that support an environment for optimal health at the spiritual level.

Acknowledgment of Our Dependence on a Higher Power

Human beings are subject to the higher laws of nature, just like all phenomena in the universe. Recognition of our human boundaries opens our body and mind to Divine healing forces. Acknowledgment of our dependence opens the pathway for us to achieve spiritual maturity.

It is fascinating when we stop to think about the awesome complexity and balance of the universe. The more we explore and learn, the greater our appreciation for how much more there is to know. By following the laws of nature and trusting in the Creator who governs our universe, health is enabled beyond today's limited comprehension.

Love for Our Fellow Man

Love's mysterious healing energy uplifts us personally and improves our social relationships. It is powerful enough to "heal" our entire planet.

Daily Exercise of Our Spiritual Self

Practice makes perfect. It is important to regularly spend some quiet time to awaken our inner mind and spiritual self. Daily Bible study, prayer, and service to others are among the most powerful spiritual calisthenics known to man. With the daily distractions of today's frenetic pace, daily focus on our spiritual side will guard our immune system against the ever-increasing health challenges we face.

Learning from Nature

Nature teaches many lessons regarding nurturing and healthy living. By observing, studying, and applying the powerful laws of nature to our lives, our spiritual enrichment overcomes the boundaries and mysteries of physical limitations.

An Active Prayer Life

Throughout history, civilizations have demonstrated their natural propensity to communicate with a higher power. Prayer is legendary for its powerful healing influences. Throughout our recorded history, it has healed many conditions with its powerfully effective life force. Many things may seem right in the light of human knowledge but ultimately lead to disappointing results. An active prayer life opens our minds and hearts to the Source of all knowledge, wisdom, and health.

Our spiritual nature differentiates us from every other living thing on our planet. Many of us instinctively feed ourselves with the healing energy assimilated through spiritual things. The spiritual element is the most powerful element of our being, one that allows us to transcend the limitations of all known human knowledge to receive a mysteriously perfect and lasting gift of health.

In my naturopathic practice, I like to start a personalized health plan for each client with the first and most important element. Namely, I instruct a client in this way: "Spend special time in prayer daily. God can do everything, and when we pray to Him, we can do everything He can do!"

Trust and reliance on a loving, powerful God give the ability to enjoy a healthful lifestyle. Complete belief in God permits Him to fill our lives with outrageous and radiant health!

Eight Laws of Health: SUMMARY AND CONCLUSIONS

The integrated and comprehensive use of the eight laws of health makes up the most powerful health-enhancing system known to man. These time-honored principles are the implementation of the original medicine concept. As important as nutrition or a proper diet is in relation to good health, it can be quite meaningless if we are not practicing all eight natural laws of health.

The effectiveness of all other methods of maintaining and enhancing health should be evaluated on the basis of their promotion of these foundational laws of health. We should be thankful for the power of these simple laws, apply them to ourselves, and then lovingly share them with our family, friends, and associates for a richer and healthier society, neighborhood, and world.

Final Thoughts on Original Medicine

Original medicine draws its knowledge and inspiration from the Bible with its descriptions of a Creator, the origin of man, and the original diet. Honor and glory belong to God alone for all health since He is the Originator and Creator of all things. All human beings and their inventions, systems, power, and wisdom are subordinate to His power and wisdom.

Original medicine embraces the fact that God is the Author of the natural laws of health and has placed within our power the means for obtaining knowledge of these laws of health. Original medicine encourages putting forth the needed effort to obtain knowledge of God's laws of life and the simple means He has chosen to be employed to restore health. It is our duty to preserve our physical and mental powers in the best possible condition so that we may effectively serve our fellow man and Him. When sickness is the result of the transgression of natural law, we should seek to correct the error and then ask for the blessing of God. Those who refuse to improve the light and knowledge that have been mercifully placed within their reach are rejecting one of the means that God has granted them to promote spiritual as well as physical life.

Summary and Conclusions

Thus, man and all created things in the world were perfect in every way. There was a powerful simplicity and integrity that governed our beginnings. The natural treasures established at the dawn of humanity have withstood the test of time, even today, as the most powerful system of health, longevity, and happiness. For the prevention and reversal of disease, our best opportunity is to be in harmony with these immutable laws.

Many of the health systems today provide varying degrees of the elements of the original prescription for health and vitality. To the extent that they are in harmony with the original principles, they enjoy their greatest opportunity for effectiveness. Our health status is also amenable to these same principles and concepts. These principles are not man-made, nor has man demonstrated any ability to improve them.

The original medicine concept takes us back to our roots and encourages us to rediscover the power and simplicity of the eight wonders of the world to maximize our potential. We are made by a loving Creator who provided us everything we need from the beginning of time to enjoy a profoundly happy existence on this planet. Knowledge and application of His laws give us a standard for evaluating other health systems and modalities.

The time-honored wonders of the **original medicine** world can be summarized with the acronym:

GODSPLAN:

	Godly Trust	A belief and trust in God, the Creator
	Open Air	Fresh, pure air and it's healing qualities
	Daily Exercise	Stimulating the body's muscles, organs and systems with regular exercise
	Sunshine	The sun's healing energy
	Proper Rest	Regenerate and replenish our systemic resources with proper rest
	Lots of Water	Regenerate and replenish our systemic resources with proper rest
	Always Temperate	Temperance and self-control, leading to optimal health
	Nutrition	Living, natural, organic foods that promote the life force within us

The International Institute of Original Medicine (IIOM) Hierarchy of Healing includes the following original medicine principles.

1. Avoid all harmful factors causing or contributing to the condition.

2. Use natural, harmless, and simple remedies freely. These include air, water, sunlight, nutrition, exercise, rest, moderation, gratitude, benevolence, and trust in Divine Power.

3. Use "less harmful" remedies, such as selected natural substances and herbs, judiciously.

4. Only rarely, when all else has failed, turn to conventional drugs. Generally speaking, this should be a last resort, not the first resort.

5. Pray, thank God for His many blessings, and seek His wisdom and guidance in all things, including health and healing.

Basic Concepts and Explanation of RBTI

Origin and Basics of RBTI

The RBTI system is a powerful healing technology, unlike any tool in the allopathic or naturopathic healing modalities. This is about how the body is put together and taken apart. An equation for perfect health is central to the analysis as it provides a simple method of analyzing one person's biochemistry, assessing the loss or gain of energy, and, most importantly, providing a signpost for diet and lifestyle changes to minimize energy loss.

We are seeking the truth based strictly on a mathematical principle – not on perceived truth, not on generally accepted truth, not on a financially beneficial truth, and not on a convenient theory.

Dr. Carey Reams, in 1931, discovered a testing system that measured how far away from **"biochemical balance"** the human body could be. Reams formed a theory called **"Reams Biological Theory of Ionization" (RBTI)**. **This mathematical measuring tool** indicates the body's biochemical position and determines where in the body attention is needed to bring it to an optimal state in relation to health.

The non-invasive biochemical testing will reveal the practical steps to regain optimal health. A measurement of residues and components in samples of urine and saliva indicates if the body is out of balance and enables a practitioner to suggest a program of dietary mineral supplementation and lifestyle changes to access vibrant health.

The RBTI Equation is a signpost that shows;

- How far away from **"biochemically perfect"** a person is positioned.
- The direction that is needed for a person to gain perfect health.
- Whether the body is cooperating in improving or not.
- Whether or not the body is improving from the program's suggestions.

Dr. Carey Reams always identified himself as a biophysicist. After first making the discovery in 1931, he launched his vision of natural energy-based health, first in agriculture by producing high-mineral foods, and then, in 1968, as a system of healing in a world of harsh drugs and unnecessary surgery.

Reams devised a formula that speaks to **HEALTH** as opposed to disease. He found that when certain factors of a person's urine and saliva are within easily maintained parameters, physical illness is impossible. An individual's results are used to create a personal wellness program specially designed to address the imbalances in their body with common sense, proper hydration, diet, movement, and nutritional supplements.

Reams commenced teaching his science and methods in the 60s and 70s and passed to his rest in 1985. He had wonderful success in supporting people, often with life-threatening illnesses, to live healthy lives; however, all the attention eventually brought the guise of the medical industry, and he eventually suffered the wrath for not conforming to the established disease industry. Reams was a brilliant mathematician who could identify patterns in numbers and conversed with Einstein on the mathematics of energy. A man of great faith, a biochemist, an officer in the army, and a husband and father to a beautiful family, he spent time behind bars for treating people without a medical license. His crime was teaching individuals the correct diet and hydration regimes to achieve health.

One of his dreams was that his science would be shared and taught to every household around the world so that many people could experience the wonder of vibrant physical, emotional, mental, and spiritual health.

This is part of his vision.

Reams' frequently stated maxims included:

- "The equation is a way of formulating a better diet for ONE person."
- "Go by the numbers."
- "Trust the numbers; the numbers don't lie. "
- "Why guess when you can be sure? "
- "We don't live off the food we eat; we live off the energy created by the minerals in the food we eat. "

As a mathematical genius, Carey Reams was very familiar with Einstein's energy equation and understood its significance. During his meeting at Princeton University with Albert Einstein, he once chided him, saying, "You taught us how to take matter apart, but how do we put it back together again?"

Einstein immediately shot back, "That's for you to find out."

And so, Reams completed the assignment by producing the formula for Perfect Health for all biological life – the Theory of Ionization – a universal law placed into theory that he scribed into a mathematical form.

The Mathematical Formula for Perfect Health

The Equation in a simplified form is: **PERFECT HEALTH =**

$$PH = CS + \underset{\text{Brix}}{1.5} \quad \underset{\text{pH}}{6.4/6.4} \quad \underset{\text{Salt}}{6\text{-}7C} \quad \underset{\text{Cellular Debris}}{.04M} \quad \underset{\text{Ureas}}{3/3}$$

PH	= Perfect Health
CS	= Common Sense
Brix	= % of total sugars
pH	= potential for Hydrogen (alkalinity or acidity)
Salt	= % of total salts
Cellular Debris	= amount of dead and dying cells as parts per million
Ureas	= Nitrogen nitrate and Ammonia nitrate

From this equation, it is possible to:
- Determine hydration, foods, and supplements that should be added to or eliminated from an individual's diet.
- Demonstrate how complex issues of ill health and lack of optimum performance can be minimized.

Symptoms can be easily and quickly relieved by the information gained through "the numbers." For example, when a client's pH is too fast or too slow, or the carbs and salts are too high or too low, the body will have difficulty absorbing all of the minerals and nutrients needed to maintain optimum health. The further the numbers are away from perfect, the greater the symptoms.

Being "out of balance" will result in many different symptoms and conditions:
- Disease
- Hormonal imbalance
- Anxiety
- Depression
- Irritable bowel
- Aches and pains
- Headaches and
- Any condition less than optimal health.

Using the correct calcium for an individual's body is often the quickest way to re-balance the biochemistry. A similar system is used in naturally based agricultural practices to enhance crop yields with healthier fruit, vegetables, and even livestock. Developed and refined over many years, it has been successfully used to assist the better health of babies, children, teenagers, adults, and sportspeople to assist in performance and recovery from injury.

The test is a true real-time mathematical analysis of what is taking place within the electro-biochemical structure of the human body's cells, tissues, and organs. It reveals the intricate cause and effect of the physiological dysfunctional patterns demonstrated through urine and saliva analysis. The individual may or may not be aware of the dysfunctions the tests may highlight. More importantly, the BE Analysis will reveal a lifestyle program for each person to reverse or minimize the dysfunctional patterns.

Healthcare professionals and personal users can stay in close communication, sharing their results from anywhere in the world, in real-time, on smartphones, laptops, or desktop computers. The numbers will reveal steps to take to improve health scores immediately, such as:
- How much water to consume,
- What juices and fluids to use, and when,
- What foods to eliminate or avoid,
- What type of mineral supplements to use and when,
- What type of vitamins, herbs, and enzymes to use and when, and
- What type of ancillary treatments to use to better the "numbers.

The benefits are endless when individuals are ready to investigate the causes rather than the symptoms.

Summary of RBTI Analysis:

- Is based on a mathematical equation to measure the body's chemistry and, through specific diet and lifestyle changes, enables one to achieve optimum health.
- Creates a specific diet for a person based on their biochemistry.
- Deals with the mathematics and chemistry of a gain or loss of energy through accurate analysis of urine and saliva.
- Manages the cause and effect of an illness due to mineral deficiency, the primary mineral being calcium.
- Handles the cleansing of the body by improving diet, lifestyle changes, and drinking the correct amount of clean, pure, distilled water.
- Recognizes the cause of the malfunction of vital organs as insufficient or incorrect mineral types in the diet needed to replace the worn-out cells.
- Maintains that harmful bacteria and fungus are **NOT** the cause of disease but do complicate an already weakened biochemical status.
- Offers a powerful, commonsense approach to nutrition and optimal health.

Now, let's look at each of the seven numbers in the formula.

CARBOHYDRATES

1.5

Oxygen and the Blood, Available Energy, Natural Sweeteners

In his book *Biological Ionization as Applied to Human Nutrition*, Dr. Alexander Beddoe wrote, "The Carbohydrate number has the greatest effect on the overall conscious and subconscious feeling of well-being than any other number in the equation."[1] In this chapter, you will learn how simple it is to understand your "sugar level" after digestion and manage it to enable optimum energy.

CARBOHYDRATES – Total Sugars – Brix

Total Carbohydrates, which are often referred to as "carbs," sugar, and/or brix, is a percentage indication of total carbohydrates, which includes both natural and processed sugars.

A perfect reading is 1.5 when all other numbers are perfect.

The Healing Range is 1.2 – 2.0 when all other numbers are in the Healing Range.

Carbohydrates are sugar molecules, and the total sugar measurement in RBTI is obtained with a Refractometer and measured in Brix. **It is important to remember that no carbohydrate number is perfect unless all other numbers are perfect.**

One of the primary functions of carbohydrates is to provide your brain and your body with enough energy to sustain life, and this energy is provided in the form of glucose. Glucose is necessary to support your body's everyday needs and performance. However, if the level is too low or too high, the body's ability to convert energy is compromised. Some carbs last longer than others. Some carbs come from processed sugar, and others from food and fluids.

Total carbohydrates in the urine indicate the body's ability to digest and utilize carbohydrates to maintain consistent energy efficiently. Any variation moving away from Range A or the *Healing Range* is an indication of difficulty holding optimum blood sugar balance. An imbalance affects the ability to sustain energy and causes unnecessary stress to the body. This can lead to

---

[1] Beddoe, A. (2008). *Biological Ionization as Applied to Human Nutrition*. Advanced Ideal Institute. p47

fatigue, cravings, and poor dietary control, as well as many other symptoms such as anxiety, depression, and addictions.

Important Brix Facts

Sugar is only one component of Brix. Brix is a measurement of the percentage of total dissolved solids in a given weight of fluid, i.e., fruit or vegetable juices, urine samples, etc. In relation to URINE as a post-digestion result, Brix includes the number of total sugars that remain as waste.

A too-high or too-low Brix reading indicates a reduction in the body's ability to produce energy,

While Brix equals the percentage of sucrose, it is also a summation of the weight of sucrose, fructose, vitamins, minerals, amino acids, proteins, hormones, and other solids in one hundred units, grams/ounces, pounds, or kilos of any particular juice or fluid.

Regarding food and juices, high Brix content means high mineral content. **Brix varies directly with food quality**; e.g., a poor, sour-tasting grape from worn-out soil can test 8 percent or less Brix. On the other hand, a full-flavored, delicious grape grown in rich, fertile soil can test 24 percent or higher in Brix.

Carbs provide your body with energy. One of the primary functions of carbohydrates is to provide your body and brain with energy to sustain life.

Total carbohydrates in the urine indicate the body's ability to efficiently digest and utilize carbohydrates to maintain consistent energy. Any variation from the ideal zone is an indication of difficulty holding optimum blood sugar balance. An imbalance affects the ability to sustain energy and causes unnecessary stress to the body. This can lead to fatigue, cravings, and poor dietary control, as well as many other symptoms such as anxiety, depression, and addictions.

NATURAL SUGARS

Once a person discovers the right food for their body, this valuable information will remain with them for the rest of their life.

Natural sugars from natural foods are sweet because of their high mineral quality and quantity. The type of mineral in a sweet apple is different than in a sweet pear.

Our body needs a large variety of foods. The different flavors are made up of different minerals. Different foods with different flavors – bitter, salty, sour, astringent, sweet, pungent (e.g., chili), and savory – have different minerals and different volumes of minerals.

There are times when you will need to raise the carb level with natural sugars because the carb level has fallen too low. Learn which natural sweeteners move your numbers up or down. It is important to understand that what is good for some will not work for others, and we should find out which one works for us individually. Not all people will respond the same.

Natural sugars include but are not limited to:
- Brown Sugar
- Black Strap Molasses – unsulphured
- Grandma's Molasses – unsulphured
- Date Sugar
- Maple Syrup
- Sorghum
- Coconut Sugar
- Agave Nectar
- Rice Syrup
- Honey

SYMPTOMS THAT OCCUR WITH BOTH HIGH AND LOW SUGAR

The further away from the Healing Range (1.2 to 2.0 percent), whether the reading is too high or too low, **the lower the oxygen level will be in the blood**. This is known as a biochemical form of choking.

Results can be influenced by gender, age, height, weight, occupation, and personal religious beliefs (e.g., religious practice that requires fasting with no water). It is important to look for all environmental influences (e.g., indoor air pollution, smoke-filled rooms, radon, exposure to pesticides, herbicides, medications, supplements, etc.) when looking for a cause. Symptoms can all be managed by proper hydration and sugar/carb consumption.

Too High or **Too Low** levels of sugar compromise oxygen getting to the brain and serve as a component in causing mineral deficiencies in the liver. The further the numbers are away from perfect, the less oxygen is available, causing:

- Tension
- Brain fog
- Anxiousness
- Light-headedness
- Forgetfulness
- Memory loss (both short and long-term)
- Headaches
- Vision issues

It is often asked what the difference is between measuring glucose levels in blood and measuring total carbohydrates in urine.

— Or —

Is the blood glucose reading the same as the sugar reading from the urine?

Urine is produced after blood is filtered through the kidneys. The Refractometer measures all sugars and carbohydrates in the urine, both simple and complex.

The reading from the refractometer is a post-digestion reading and as urine collects in the bladder, usually for at least 2 to 4 hours. It is an average of all sugars eliminated over that time that the body or digestion is dealing with.

A blood glucose reading is an indicator at the point in time of collection. That reading can change very quickly.

Blood glucose tests measure only one sugar – glucose. The blood glucose and the urine carbohydrates will differ because of the incomplete metabolism of carbohydrates indigestion. This, in turn, results from an ongoing lack of minerals for the liver. The pancreas's ability to effectively coordinate with the liver in balancing blood carbohydrates is upset. Acidosis results from carbohydrate problems due to incomplete metabolism of carbs, lipids, and proteins and loss of production of bicarbonate by the pancreas.

Total Carbohydrates in Summary

Total "Carbs" is a percentage indication of total carbohydrates, which includes both natural and processed sugars.

A perfect reading is 1.5 when all other numbers are perfect.

Healing Range is 1.2 – 2.0 when all other numbers are in the Healing Range.

Carbs, like the other six numbers, have direct links to each other. It is the interrelationship patterns of all seven numbers that describe an individual's body chemistry.

In combination with the Salts reading, Carb readings are a direct indication of the hydration/dehydration state.

Apart from more technical aspects of body function, Carb readings show the efficiency with which oxygen is carried to all organs in the body.

The Carb reading indicates levels of energy directly related to emotional, mental, and physical health. A result will indicate levels of stable or unstable energy and shows an effect on moods and behavior.

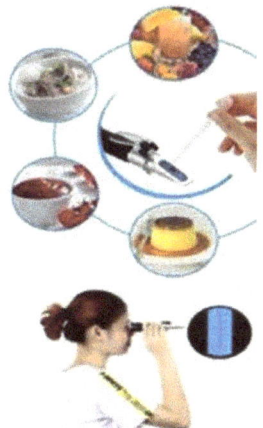

pH

6.4/6.4

Digestion, Liver Bile, Calciums

THE HEALING RANGE FOR BOTH URINE AND SALIVA IS 6.4

The pH reading is not a measure of the amount of acids or alkalines; it's a measure of resistance between acids and alkalines. By the resistance, we can tell whether one has too much, too little, or just enough calciums and what is needed to create or sustain proper resistance levels.

For human body chemistry, a perfect reading for both Urine and Saliva pH is 6.4 when all other numbers are perfect.

The Healing Range for both urine and saliva pH is 6.2 – 6.6 when all other numbers are in the Healing Range.

A scale of pH values is used as a basis for comparison with a test sample. The scale is set from 0 to 14, with 7 as the neutral or midpoint. When this scale was set up, it was based on two reference substances – pure sulfuric acid and pure calcium.

Pure sulfuric acid represents the extreme acid or cationic end of the scale, with a pH of 00. Pure calcium represents the extreme on the other end, which is anionic or basic, with a pH of 14.

In pure sulfuric acid, the electrical energy can travel at the speed of light because there is very little resistance. In pure calcium, the electrical energy travels very slowly because of very high resistance.

Pure calcium is considered a nonconductor of electrical currents relative to the pH scale. The anions that rotate around the cation in the calcium atom move as slowly as possible for them to move and still make the element calcium.

Energy loss is first picked up in the urine and saliva pH. The more the urine and saliva pHs move away from Range A, the more they indicate that the digestive enzymes are becoming too diluted and weak. This weakness of digestion and its enzymes is primarily due to the lack of one very important mineral, calcium, and occurs in both the cationic and the anionic direction.

While studying the science of foods, Dr. Reams discovered that the ideal pH level for all biological life was 6.40. That is, the food enters and exits at 6.4 pH and therefore incurs "the LEAST amount of ENERGY LOSS." When the pH is 6.4, all Energy is directed toward creating new cells and eliminating dead and dying cells.

Science of pH Behind RBTI

Ultimately, the entire body's electro-chemistry depends on the body's ability to properly digest, release, and process energy from food converted into energy that can be used to build and maintain cells of tissues and organs on the proper frequency. **Frequency is defined as "the periodic motion of electrons around atoms of molecules.** Specifically, it refers to the time for one revolution or period. It is the common denominator or energy exchange ratio necessary for a living system to continue to function properly."[2]

While studying the science of foods, Dr. Reams discovered that the perfect pH level for all biological life was 6.40. That is, when food enters and exits at 6.4 pH, it incurs "the LEAST amount of ENERGY LOSS." When the pH is 6.4, all energy is directed toward the creation of new cells and the elimination of dead and dying cells.

Reams taught that we don't live on food, but rather, **we live off the energy provided by the minerals in the food**. For minerals to be used by the human body, they must be put on the **frequency** of the human body by combining them in the right amounts and proportions for ionization for cellular replacement.

In Choose Life or Death, Reams writes, "The pH reading is not a measure of the amount of acids or alkalines, it's a **measure of resistance between acids and alkalines**. By the resistance, we can tell whether we have too much or too little calciums, or which calciums are enough and of which ones ... are too much. It is not a quantitative measure, it's a **measure of resistance**."[3]

Even though 7 is the neutral midpoint on the pH scale, it doesn't relate to efficient digestion. Efficient digestion has everything to do with the energy resulting from the correct balance of anions and cations in the food we eat. Reams stated that **a wide variety of foods in the diet is essential for a balanced biochemistry**. If nothing else, **this rule alone, along with correct hydration, will promote improved health and vitality.**

---

[2] Beddoe, A. (2008). *Biological Ionization as Applied to Human Nutrition*. Advanced Ideal Institute. p5

[3] Reams, C. (1978). *Choose Life or Death*. Harrison, Arkansas, New Leaf Press, Inc., p16.

Simply put, during digestion, when the opposing ions come together or clash, that spark is the element of energy produced. If the ratio of ions is imbalanced, digestion speed is affected, and ineffective digestion occurs.

For example, if there are **Too Many cations**, the digestion will move **Too Fast,** and the pH will be a low number; e.g., 5.2. This means digestion will be compromised in the assimilation of certain minerals and vitamins needed by the body. A low pH may cause hunger not long after meals due to fast digestion. If there are **Too Many anions**, the digestion will be moving **Too Slow,** and the pH will be a high number, e.g., 7.2. In this case, digestion is again compromised, and the assimilation of needed minerals and vitamins will not take place.

The body is in the business of producing energy – energy to stay alive first and then energy to do the things we love to do. Providing the body with the exact levels of minerals, nutrients, and hydration that serve energy requirements is the ultimate goal.

The **urine pH** is extremely important, as it is an indication of how well your body **has** digested and assimilated the nutrients from food and supplements. You may be wasting your money consuming foods and supplements that you can't efficiently absorb if your pH is too acid or too alkaline.

The **saliva pH** indicates the pressure on the liver. Dr. Reams said it was a reading of the strength of the liver bile and how it relates to the body's ability to begin the digestive process in the mouth—an indication of **what's going to happen** in digestion. Calcium is the element most highly needed by the body.

pH guides us to recognize which Calciums your body may be lacking. Having the right balance of all the Calciums in your body serves many roles. Amongst others, it will help ensure the correct production of enzymes for digestion and support the assimilation of all other nutrients, minerals, and vitamins. There are numerous benefits to list. They include correcting any imbalances that can renew energy levels, assist in correcting weight, help in calming the body, mind, and spirit, and cope with stress more easily.

The further away from 6.4 the pH of the urine or saliva is, in either direction, can be a sign of cause of illness and disease. Reams stated that "all disease begins with a mineral deficiency." "The liver is where mineral deficiency occurs." If ignored, an imbalanced pH can affect your blood and oxygen-carrying capacity and pancreatic function, along with all cellular function.

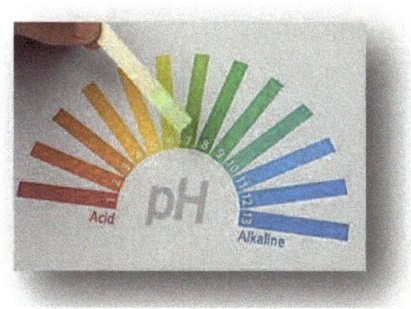

CONDUCTIVITY/SALTS
6C to 7C
Membranes, Osmotic Pressure, Blood Viscosity, Electric Current, Electrolytes

The Conductivity/Salts number reveals the amount of electricity available for conductance in the body. By measuring salts, we are looking at levels of conductance (salts carry the electricity), which tell us how well the brain is delivering communication to the liver, the gut, and the rest of the body. If the numbers are in the Healing Range, the messages will get through with ease and minimal energy loss.

Perfect is 6.5C when all other numbers are perfect.

6C – 12C = the Healing Range when all other numbers are in the Healing Range. This range is reflected in blue shading on the Range and Zone Chart.

Besides serving as the conductor of electricity, salts perform other vital functions in the body, like the destruction of worms and parasites and the purification of cellular waste. Our emphasis will be on ionization and salt as a conductor of electricity throughout the body.

The conductivity reading is derived from at least 48 different varieties of salts within two main groups found in the body. The two main groups are:

- **Chloride Salts**, such as calcium chloride, potassium chloride, sodium chloride, etc.; and
- **Non-chloride salts**, such as insulin, urea, nitrate nitrogen, and ammonia nitrogen.

There are many different types of chloride salts. In fact, most salts are chloride, and when you get a salt substitute, it simply means that the salt is not the same as sodium chloride table salt. The substitute, however, is still a chloride salt; it's just not sodium chloride.

Excess or depletion of salt will cause many unwanted lifestyle disease issues. Salt readings that are not in balance can affect electrolyte levels and hydration efficiency and cause deterioration in the function of nerve and muscle systems, ultimately affecting optimal health. Salt levels that impact the nervous system with too much or too little electrical force drive the vital organs and body systems in ways that can cause hypertension, hyperactivity, and nervousness. The detrimental effects of salts tend to be AGE-related, particularly high salts. Generally, the higher the salt reading and the longer the time, the more damage is being done and the greater the stress on the heart and vascular system of the body. Remember, the further away from the perfect numbers, the lower the reserve energy.

High Salts

High Salts impact the nervous system with **Too Much electrical force**, causing loss of elasticity in veins and arteries. High salts draw moisture out of cartilage. The body systems are being overstimulated and shorted out, causing energy loss, inflammation, and congestion. High salt levels are primarily due to high salt intake, improper hydration, or a combination of both. Enough cannot be said regarding high-salt diets and the ensuing damage they cause to biochemistry. High salt content and ratios in processed foods are extremely detrimental to the body and are an indication of a potential salting-out effect.

When looking at heart and blood health, high Conductivity/Salts readings are a major indicator/warning of a potential heart health problem! Pressure in the vascular system results in high-frequency delivery of communication from the brain to soft tissue organs. This causes a breakdown of tissue in the smooth muscles of the body, including the brain, heart, kidneys, and lungs. It also can cause excess cholesterol in the vascular system, show the effects of atherosclerosis, and draw moisture from cartilage. High salt levels can also cause hemorrhoids, varicose veins, intestinal polyps, diverticulitis, and high blood pressure.

If the soil has a high salt content, the land struggles to produce fruits, vegetables, and grass for feedlots. The land becomes barren. The same principle applies to the body. **ONE WORD CAN DESCRIBE HIGH SALTS – INTENSE!**

Low Salts

When one's salts are **Too Low**, messages necessary for communication from the brain to various parts of the body are delayed and ineffective. Low salts impact the nervous system by providing **Too Little electrical force** in the body. Low salts result in the body's system not functioning at an optimum level. Low salts may cause individuals to become increasingly slow, both mentally and physically, causing them to have difficulty with coordination. Low salts can also cause tiredness, fatigue, anxiousness, and disconnection.

CELLULAR DEBRIS

.04M

Rate of Cell Replacement, Kidney Function, Protein Deterioration

The Cellular Debris test is a general count of cellular particles in the urine due to cellular exchange. Every cell in the human adult body should be exchanged within a six-month period. If it takes an adult human longer than six months to replace all cells, it shortens the life span.

0.04M = perfect when all other numbers are perfect.

4M = the Healing Range when all other numbers are in the Healing Range.

This number is most relevant as a healing indicator. It gives us a clear view of the functioning of the kidneys in removing waste and toxins from the body system.

If all other numbers are not perfect, then a cell debris reading of .04M or lower means that cellular debris (dead cells) is being blocked somewhere. In other words, if any of the other numbers are off or out of the "A" Range, it means there is a greater density of dead cells (rapid cell die-off), so your cell debris number should also be higher than "A" Range to show that all those extra dead cells are being thrown out by the body. So, to recap, if your other numbers are off, it indicates greater cell die-off.

If your cell debris number is in the "A" range or lower, it indicates that the dead cells (toxic waste) are blocked somewhere and not being kicked out of the body. In the case of healing, you actually want this number to be high when any of the other numbers are off.

Aging or Healing?

Several things can be deduced from the cell debris number.

First, the higher the cell debris number on your initial test, the faster your body is breaking down and aging.

Second, when the cell debris number is high, and the rest of the numbers are away from the "A" range, it shows that nature is cooperating in the healing process.

These two statements may seem to contradict one another, so let me explain. Whether healthy or not, your body dumps old, worn-out cells. That's what it's supposed to do. That means it's cooperating. It may be throwing them out too fast (aging), but at least it's throwing them out.

Now, whether you replace those cells with healthy cells is another story, and this determines whether you call this process of cell die-off either aging or healing.

If you are not replacing them with healthy cells, then you are aging and probably prematurely. However, if you are replacing these cells with healthy cells, you are healing.

Third, if the cell debris number is lower than the perfect reading and the rest of the numbers are away from the "A" range, it is an indication that the body is having trouble removing dead cells, which could be due to dead cell buildup somewhere in the body.

This would be a good indication for a detox. In fact, detoxing is a major part of the RBTI program.

And fourth, if the cell debris number is less than the perfect reading and the rest of the numbers are moving toward the "A" range, it could be an indication that the body and possibly the kidneys are not completely cooperating.

While healing, it is not unusual to see this number jump much higher than 4M. This only shows that the body is able and willing to get rid of dead cell debris when given the chance and that there is healthy kidney function. This is part of the healing process.

UREAS

3/3

Protein Utilization, Nitrogen, and Ammonia Nitrate Salts

Ureas are a result of undigested protein and the last two numbers in the equation. They represent the two kinds of nitrogen found in our body chemistry: Nitrate Nitrogen and Ammonia Nitrogen. The Nitrate Nitrogen is ANIONIC, usually BLUE (think of the Sky), and recorded on the top. The Ammonia Nitrogen is CATIONIC, usually YELLOW and/or BROWN (think of the Earth), and recorded on the bottom.

3 over 3 is perfect for both urea numbers when all other numbers are perfect.

A combined total of 12 to 19 are in the Healing Range (as long as both numbers are no more than two digits apart and all other numbers are in the Healing Range). The ureas are higher in the Healing Range because to heal; the body must rid itself of toxic dead and dying cells before new cells can be built.

Nitrate Nitrogen comes from excess proteins, both properly and improperly digested proteins, in daily food. **Ammonia Nitrogen is the product of the breakdown of cells** along with other breakdown products of cell metabolism and the tissues themselves due to the aging process. These numbers are part of an anionic-cationic relationship or ratio. They influence the electromagnetic picture that develops from the ratio of differentials and represents energy being lost from the system. If **Too Low** or **Too High**, they're showing **energy loss** in the body.

Nitrate Nitrogen and **Ammonia Nitrogen** are either insoluble or soluble salts. Nitrate Nitrogen is an insoluble protein that has not been digested and should be washed out of the body with hydration. It can also be digested protein that is not utilized by the body because it isn't on the same frequency as the human body. If the insoluble protein stays in the body longer than three days, it is released as a soluble salt.

The core of every biological cell is nitrogen, and protein is nitrogen. In human adults, biological cells should be exchanged every six months. If they are not exchanged, they become **sick cells**, i.e., **Delta or Carcinoma cells**, as opposed to healthy cells.

Certain things happen within a cell that begins to wear out. A space appears within the nitrogen core of the cell—a gas forms within the space, which causes the core to expand a little. Water displaces the gas in the core and moves the nitrogen core out of the cell. At this point, the cell is degenerated and should be cast out into the bloodstream and filtered out of the body through the kidneys.

If the results of this cellular protein breakdown in the body are removed within three days, it is eliminated as an insoluble protein.

The insoluble form of urea shows up as Nitrate or Ammonia Nitrogen and does not affect the heart. If a cell that contains urea in the insoluble form stays in the body for longer than three days after being released from its location, it will turn into the soluble form of urea and show up as Nitrate or Ammonia Nitrogen on the urea test. Soluble urea, as a salt, is most damaging to the heart and will stimulate the heart to beat harder or stronger than it should. This is one of the reasons for drinking pure distilled water systematically throughout the day. When Delta or Carcinoma (sick) cells are exchanged and removed in the insoluble form of urea, they will not turn into the soluble form.

In the digestion process, amino acids combine to form proteins. When the urine and saliva numbers are outside of the Healing Range, improper digestion results in the release of amino acids that are NOT on the frequency of the body. Simply put, the liver cannot use those amino acids to make energy-building blocks for the body and convert them into non-toxic insoluble urea. However, that non-toxic conversion of unusable protein only stays non-toxic for a few days. After 72 hours, it begins to break down into soluble urea salts of Nitrate Nitrogen. In large quantities, this is unhealthy for the body.

Combined Ureas

Combined Ureas are simply **the two urea results added together**. The higher the Combined Urea numbers, the more wastes are retained, and the likelihood of toxicity building throughout the whole body through poor digestion and lack of elimination of protein breakdown in the body.

When Salt/Conductivity levels are high, >35C, the body experiences a salting out effect. This will further aggravate the urea number.

Together, the urea numbers are part of an anionic-cationic relationship or ratio. When **Too High**, these numbers represent energy being lost from the system. When **Too Low**, they're showing not enough energy entering into the body.

Combined Ureas are a factor in the line of least resistance and the resulting symptomatic effects produced by such. Digestion either provides usable energy on the frequency of the body, or it provides unusable energy that is not on the frequency of the body and can become toxic.

Effects of Digestion on Ureas

When food enters digestion, resistance is encountered. This is a chemical reaction that takes place between the digestive enzymes and the food. In other words, a chemical pressure is applied to the food to take it apart and convert it into simpler forms – matter (cells), heat, and electricity.

When water, oxygen, appropriate foods, and the right kind of calciums are properly supplied to the body, digestion will apply the correct amount of resistance to the food, resulting in the beginning of the proper frequency, or line of resistance, from the energy released. This properly adjusted energy can then be picked up by the liver, which will use it to create all the basic building blocks for healthy cell development.

If the amount of the resistance on the incoming food is not correct because of a lack of water, oxygen, and/or calciums in the food and the body, the matter, heat, and electricity will be released on the wrong frequency (incorrect line of resistance) – and unusable by the body.

Ureas In Children

In children, high ureas, as well as high cholesterol, may cause pains in the stomach, but it doesn't in adults. Breastfed children can have just as high urea as those who do not if the mother's urea is too high. This can cause or contribute to crib death.

Potassium and Proteins

If a pattern of protein deficiency continues long enough, a potassium deficiency will develop. The pickup of potassium by the intestines is dependent on the proper levels of nitrogen in the body (obtained from protein). Regarding the person's weight, potassium is necessary for the thyroid gland to make an emulsifying agent used in the bile for fat metabolism.

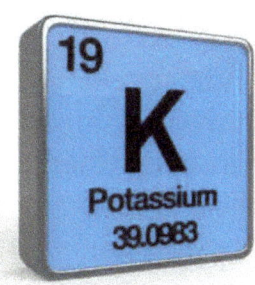

Potassium is one of the minerals that is seldom lacking in the diet; however, it can be lacking in sufficient levels in the tissues. This means that even though the amount of potassium in the foods eaten is sufficient, the body is unable to get it out of the digestion because of the way it is functioning.

Potassium is necessary for the proper function of body chemistry in all human life. It is a vital part of the electrical impulse response of nerves, as well as the nutrient fluid exchange inside (intracellular) and outside (extracellular) of the cell.

Next to calcium and phosphate, potassium is the chief mineral in the makeup of the brain's molecular structure. When potassium in the brain is lacking, there is a highly increased danger of the formation of brain tumors.

The objective is to allow nature to follow the line of least resistance and cause the body to start accepting potassium. If the body begins to accept potassium, the ureas will rise above a total of 12, and this implies that the body's chemistry is responding to the diet. If the ureas do not go above 12, the body chemistry is not responding, and the potassium is not being accepted. The brain is the organ that needs potassium the most in the body.

Remember that the urea numbers 3/3 are perfect when all other numbers are perfect. Human body chemistry will not return to perfect suddenly unless God does supernatural healing. The liver must be rebuilt before the numbers are able to come into the Perfect Range.

As nature is rebuilding the liver, it is throwing out the old and building new cells. The goal for the ureas during this rebuilding stage is to keep the combined total in the Healing Range between 12 and 19. When the liver is rebuilt, the Urea and Cell Debris numbers will come down together.

People who are very potassium deficient should eat potassium-rich food every day. One of the best sources of potassium is hominy. It comes in cans, and there is yellow and white hominy. If it is not available in your area in the markets, ask your grocer to special order a case of each for you. The hominy is made by soaking whole-grain corn in lye potassium hydroxide. Be sure to rinse it well before eating it.

Another source of potassium for those who are not overweight is bananas. If overweight, do not eat bananas – use the hominy. Here is a tip for buying bananas: when the banana plant gets ready to produce the banana, it sends an equal amount of potassium into each finger (banana); so, the large and small bananas have the same amount of potassium in them. Therefore, buying small bananas is more economical. Another source of potassium is sardines and tortillas. Two of the richest sources of potassium that are the most available for the body are Algazim and Min Col.

Thyroxine is manufactured by the pancreas, and as it reaches the thyroid gland, potassium is added to it. This then becomes the soap that regulates the ratio of fat and lean tissue in the body. When potassium is unavailable to the thyroid gland, there is not enough soap produced to dissolve the fats and oils. The thyroid then becomes underactive, and consequently, the result can be weight gain. People who are very potassium deficient should eat potassium-rich food every day.

Agriculture and Urea

Did you know that the reason leaves fall from trees in autumn is similar to why people have pectoris heart attacks? Have you ever wondered why leaves fall off trees? It has to do with nitrogen. In autumn, when the temperature begins to fall, and the air gets cooler, the nitrogen from the air permeates the sap. As the nitrogen concentration in the sap is increased, the sap becomes too thick and cannot flow into the stem of the leaf from the branch. So, the leaf will dry up and fall off.

In the body, if the nitrogen concentration in the blood gets high enough, it will get thicker so that the heart pumps harder to move the thicker blood. If it gets too high, the heart will spasm and cease to function. That is the cause of a pectoris heart attack. It can be preceded by aching and pain in the left arm.

In agriculture, magnesium will release nitrogen from the soil, unit for unit, pound for pound. In the body, Dolomite, which is calcium oxide and magnesium oxide, is used to release excess nitrogen. The calcium oxide of dolomite is not available to the system, but magnesium will tie up the excess nitrogen and prevent it from becoming urea.

GO BY YOUR NUMBERS ... TRUST YOUR NUMBERS

Range and Zone Chart

Ranges and Zones

RBTI Test numbers are classified into Ranges and Zones. The words "Range" and "Zone" are interchangeable as applicable to the context. Remember, high-level fatigue is a common symptom when the soluble, electrolytic ureas are elevated.

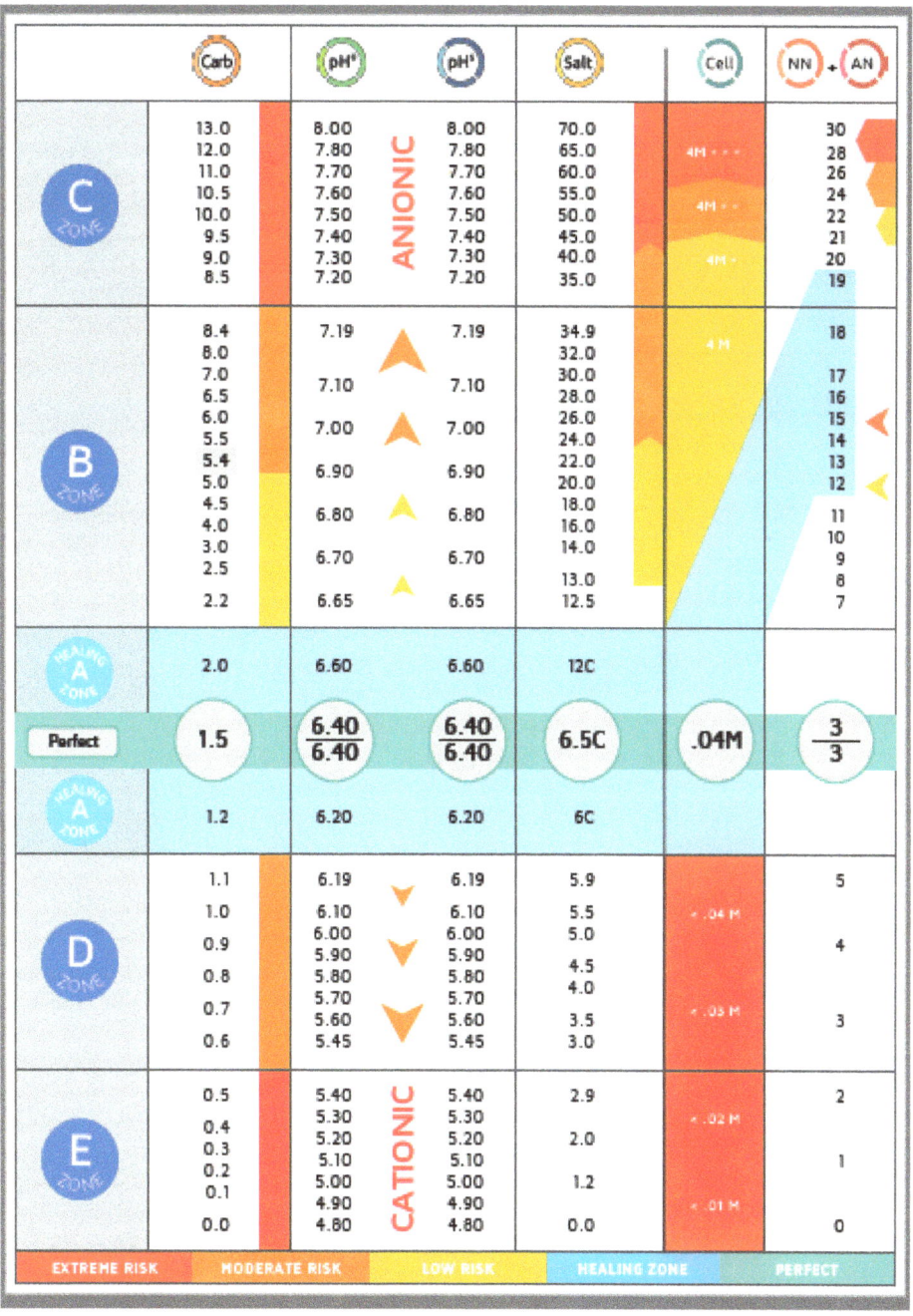

The analysis aims to locate how far away from **perfect** the numbers are and know how to bring them back within the **Healing Range** or as close to perfect for as long as possible.

It is important to remember that 80 percent of human nutrition comes from nutrients in the atmosphere. A person with perfect body chemistry is consuming the correct amounts of minerals, water, vitamins, and enzymes in the proper ratio within his or her body. This person is also getting the right amount of rest, exercise, spending time outdoors, and breathing properly – getting the maximum energy from his or her diet and the atmosphere. Reserve energy (vital force) is at its maximum for the age of the individual who is not aging too quickly because their digestion is not too fast nor too slow. The immune system is at maximum strength. **This is perfect health.**

As nutritional deficiencies occur due to improper lifestyle habits that cause wear and tear on the body, the energy level begins to drop, causing the body's chemistry numbers to move away from perfect. The greater the energy loss, the further the numbers move away from the Healing Zone; therefore, the greater the effect on one's overall health. At this time, unpleasant symptoms of all kinds may begin to affect the individual's life. When the reserve energy has dropped low enough, your physician may diagnose you with one disease or another.

The body is always attempting to return to the perfect numbers, naturally; however, if the right building blocks are not in place, the body chemistry cannot maintain balance. If the right food, right hydration, right rest, right thoughts, and right actions are not put into the body, then the body will struggle to remain in its natural state and may fall into a state of disease. Good health is natural – disease is not. The easiest way to restore "ease" to the body is to replace that which is missing so the balance can fall back into place.

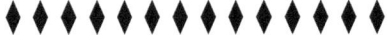

The Importance of Calcium

Dr. Reams identified almost a quarter of a million different calcium compounds. He was able to divide those into seven basic groups and consciously decided to use the word "calciums" as a means to draw attention to the wide variety.

The RBTI bio-chemical ANALYSIS will point to an alkalizing calcium, such as calcium carbonate, which can push the urinary pH up, or an acidifying calcium, such as calcium lactate, which can easily drive the pH down. On the other hand, many calciums, such as gluconate or orotate, are considered neutral because they provide the needed minerals without affecting the pH.

The heart of the problem is that modern foods are so calcium-deficient that the mineralreserve of the body falls so low that it cannot easily maintain homeostasis. This secret key is that we "should eat the widest possible diet" to bring a more balanced array of "calciums" into the body. Another part of that secret is that a wider diet brings more of the 83 other needed minerals into our system.

Although the preferred method of obtaining a sufficient mineral balance to eat higher Brix foods, and some people find they need to take calcium supplements.

According to Reams, the body needs 84 different minerals to remain healthy. The major elements needed by the body, in order of volume, are:

1. **Calcium –**. **60%** of our mineral needs are the calciums from six of the seven major groups of calcium.

2. **Phosphate – 24%** are phosphate. Without phosphates, you will not have any bones, fingernails, or teeth. It is the phosphate of calciums that forms the foundation structure for our bones and teeth.

3. **Potassium – 12%** is potassium. It is needed by the brain to communicate instructions to the body.

4. **Remaining Minerals - 4%** make up the remaining 81 minerals

The liver contains more calciums than anything else. The liver contains the greatest amount of calciums, but the next highest requirement is iron and iodine.

The heart contains a lot of calciums, but the next very essential element is arsenic.

"The main point you need to remember is that "the liver is the key organ that we work with." The liver is in the driver's seat, and when it comes to balancing the pH, there's a reason for trying to balance them quickly. If you don't give properly absorbed calciums by mouth, the body will continue to take the needed calciums from other parts of the body to sustain life.

CALCIUMS AND FEEDING THE LIVER

If you remove water and air from the human body and reduce it to ash, 80% of the body's solids are calciums. Calciums are the 5th most common mineral in both the earth's crust and in seawater, as well as by mass in the human body, where they are cellular ionic messengers with many functions as well as serving as a structural element in bone.

According to Reams, the body needs 84 different minerals to remain healthy. 60% of our mineral needs are the calciums from the six major groups of calcium; 24% are phosphate, 12% are potassium, and the remaining 4% make up the remaining 81 minerals. Calciums that are not soluble in water are hydroxide, sulfate, carbonate, and phosphate.

Different calciums will have different effects on the body, making it more acidic, alkaline, or neutral. It would be unfortunate to take a calcium supplement that aggravates an existing imbalance, so it's important to know your urine pH reading before choosing your supplement form or choose a neutral form—Reams recommended Gluconate and also mentioned that it's easy for the body to use for 're-use' when deficient, as it is in softer bone tissues; so this is also the one likely to be most deficient in some instances. The best forms of calcium will be those in the earth—natural chelates such as in Min-Col, which has lots of minerals, and second to that, in intentional composites designed for absorption such as Cal-II (which has yeast added to facilitate assimilation).

Mostly, we don't feed our body; we feed our LIVER. The liver, in turn, feeds the rest of the body. THE ANALYSIS CAN BE SUMMED UP IN THREE WORDS: **REBUILDING THE LIVER**

The Liver needs approximately 84 minerals and 20 amino acids to make the 5 to 6 billion enzymes it requires to support the human body! Deficiencies in these minerals and amino acids will significantly impact the liver's ability to perform the vast array of functions it is responsible for to deliver optimum health and vitality. Missing the "fundamental" spectrum of required calciums makes the situation worse.

Lack of calciums increases when the diversity of food goes down (e.g., when people only eat a dozen things that qualify as fresh food). Lack of calciums also increases when the frequency and quantity of fresh food that people ingest goes down. It increases when the diversity of seed types goes down (different plant forms may have different details. But when everyone eats the same kind of peas [note: there are hundreds of different seed strains for peas alone!], then that's only one option they're ever getting. Although calcium is not so affected, enzymes are often all but gone/dead by the time picked; unripe produce gets trucked to a store and eaten (and enzymes are part of the body assimilating the minerals in the food, so that can indirectly affect the calciums you get from it).

Reams was very strong on the word calciums being a plural to remind people of that importance constantly.

Reams was very strong on foods grown in decent soil, so they are nutrient-dense. For 38 years, prior to focus on human health, he was an expert in agricultural research and invented the 'Brix' measure for evaluating the nutritional density of any crop.

It is impossible to overstate the need for calcium. Still, as the ANALYSIS clearly shows, it is important to make sure that the calcium being used does not force the body into an adverse pH situation. Medically oriented physiology textbooks detail how calcium is used by the body to neutralize and dispose of harmful acidic products or by-products. The pH portion of the RBTI ANALYSIS equation allows one to estimate the mineral reserve (mostly calcium) and get a handle on the amount of available reserve energy.

RBTIOM
Putting It All Together

At the beginning of this book, we asserted that there was a powerful complementary relationship between Original Medicine and RBTI. The following table summarizes the complementary use of Original Medicine's Eight Laws of Health with the RBTI Health Analysis working in tandem – RBTIOM.

Original Medicine Remedy	RBTI Analysis Tool
Created by God to maximize human function and health	**Relationship to experiencing Perfect Health**
AIR – Genesis 1:1	**AIR**
All biological life requires oxygen	Brix measures oxygen availability and utilization
Lack of oxygen affects the function of all vital organs	The brain, which communicates to the liver via the vagus nerve, uses 20 percent of available O2
Air contains minerals and is the most important nutrient	
WATER – Genesis 1:2	**WATER**
Over 70 percent of all cells in the body Second most essential nutrient after air	The most important moderating factor for Brix, Conductivity, and Ureas
Powerful internal and external therapeutic agent	A major factor in liver functionality
	Best transporter of nutrients to cells and toxins out of cells
SUNLIGHT – Genesis 1:3	**SUNLIGHT**
Contains both visible and invisible wavelengths Stores energy in plants, nerves, and muscles	Is the best source of Vitamin D for skeletal and systemic function
Healing agent for muscles, wounds, emotions, and mind	Urine pH indicates the capacity for the assimilation of sunlight
	Powerful synthesizer of vitamins and minerals
Original Medicine Remedy	**RBTI Analysis Tool**

NUTRITION – Genesis 1:29, 3:18	**NUTRITION**
Needed for cellular development and replacement Plants provide the best sources of both quantity and ratio of nutrients and minerals for the body Herbs are God-provided medicine for systemic health and support	Best and most efficient source of mineral requirements Consuming a wide variety of foods is key to providing the 84 required minerals Analyzes individual nutrient requirements and capacities
EXERCISE – Genesis 2:15	**EXERCISE**
The human body requires movement for optimum health and vitality Helps prevention of diseases such as diabetes, blood pressure, obesity, and high cholesterol, to name a few	Provides essential movement of blood, water, and nutrients Helps to eliminate excess toxins through the skin, lymphatic system, lungs, colon, and kidneys
REST – Genesis 2:3	**REST**
Imperative for optimum health and vitality Physical, mental, emotional, and spiritual requirements	Required for all anabolic (building) activity Required for proper potassium availability required for brain
TEMPERANCE – Genesis 2:16,17	**TEMPERANCE**
Avoidance of all harmful practices and implementing good practices in moderation Underlying factor for all the laws of health	Shows whether individual numbers in the formula are **too high or too low** Helps with managing individual requirements and capacities
GODLY TRUST – Genesis 2:17	**DIVINE POWER**
We are designed (created) in the **image and likeness of God** (Genesis 1:29) Trust in Divine Power provides mental, emotional, and spiritual rest	**God's Rx** according to His original design and purpose Most effective and efficient path to maximizing **RBTI formula for Perfect Health**

In summary, there is no wisdom or knowledge that surpasses the wisdom and knowledge of God. He created us and provided all we need to sustain optimal function of **His creation** on this side of heaven until we are reunited for eternity according to **His original design** for us **in His image and likeness**.

Original Medicine is **God's Rx** for **perfect health and vitality**.

RBTI is God's faithful servant, **Carey A. Reams**, prayerfully developed, powerful, complex, and yet simple-to-use biochemical/biophysical and affordable **mathematical formula**. It shows the degree to which we live in **harmony with God's moral and natural laws of health**.

RBTIOM is the Ultimate Answer to health and Vitality:

$$PH = CS + 1.5 \quad \frac{6.4}{6.4} \quad 6.5C \quad .04M \quad \frac{3}{3}$$

PH = Perfect Health

CS = Common Sense

Perfect Health numbers are:

1.5 = Percent of Carbohydrates

6.4 = pH (for both urine and saliva)

6.5C = Conductivity/Salts (electrical current reading)

.04M = Cellular Debris (in parts per million)

3 = Ureas (for both Nitrate and Ammonia Nitrogen readings)

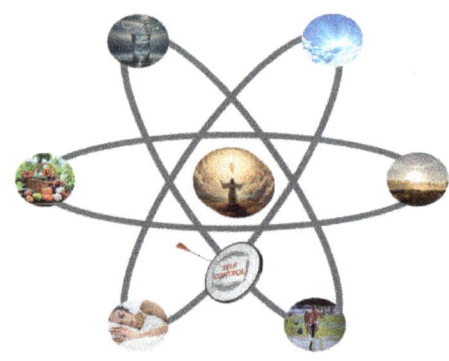

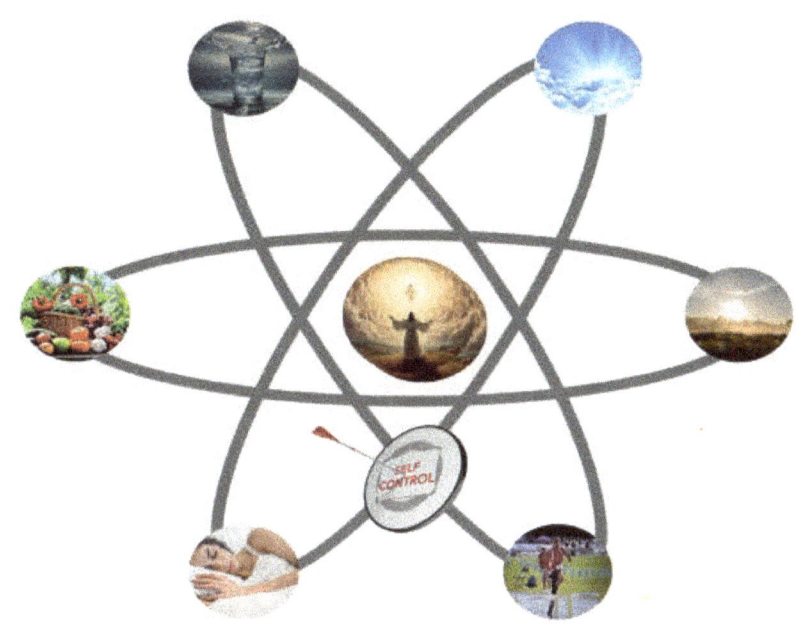

Perfect Health = 1.5 + $\dfrac{6.4}{6.4}$ + 6.5C + .04M + $\dfrac{3}{3}$

www.ingramcontent.com/pod-product-compliance
Lightning Source LLC
Chambersburg PA
CBHW041411300426
44114CB00028B/2987